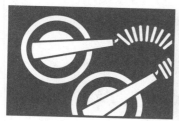

Giving Emergency Care Competently

SECOND EDITION
NURSING84 BOOKS™
SPRINGHOUSE CORPORATION
SPRINGHOUSE, PENNSYLVANIA

NURSING84 BOOKS™

NEW NURSING SKILLBOOK™ **SERIES**
Giving Emergency Care Competently
Monitoring Fluid and Electrolytes Precisely
Assessing Vital Functions Accurately
Coping with Neurologic Problems Proficiently
Reading EKGs Correctly
Combatting Cardiovascular Diseases Skillfully
Nursing Critically Ill Patients Confidently

NURSING PHOTOBOOK™ **SERIES**
Providing Respiratory Care
Managing I.V. Therapy
Dealing with Emergencies
Giving Medications
Assessing Your Patients
Using Monitors
Providing Early Mobility
Giving Cardiac Care
Performing GI Procedures
Implementing Urologic Procedures
Controlling Infection
Ensuring Intensive Care
Coping with Neurologic Disorders
Caring for Surgical Patients
Working with Orthopedic Patients
Nursing Pediatric Patients
Helping Geriatric Patients
Attending Ob/Gyn Patients
Aiding Ambulatory Patients
Carrying Out Special Procedures

NURSE'S REFERENCE LIBRARY®
Diseases
Diagnostics
Drugs
Assessment
Procedures
Definitions
Practices
Emergencies

Nursing84 DRUG HANDBOOK™

NURSING NOW™
Shock
Hypertension
Drug Interactions
Cardiac Crises
Respiratory Emergencies

NURSE'S CLINICAL LIBRARY™
Cardiovascular Disorders
Respiratory Disorders
Endocrine Disorders
Neurologic Disorders
Renal and Urologic Disorders

Giving Emergency Care Competently

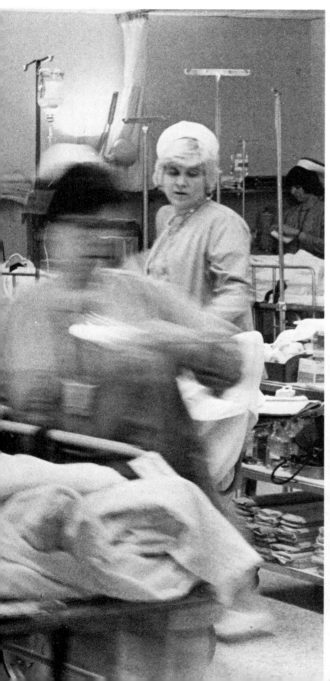
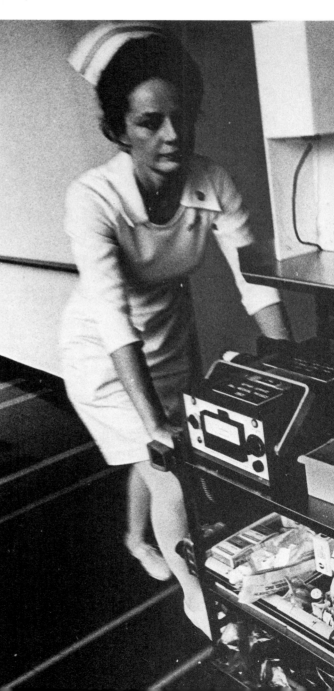

NEW NURSING SKILLBOOK™
Series
EDITORIAL PROJECT
  DIRECTOR
Jean Robinson

CLINICAL DIRECTOR
Barbara McVan, RN

ART DIRECTOR
Lisa A. Gilde

PROJECT MANAGER
Patricia R. Urosevich

**Springhouse Corporation
Book Division**
CHAIRMAN
Eugene W. Jackson

PRESIDENT
Daniel L. Cheney

VICE-PRESIDENT AND
  DIRECTOR
Timothy B. King

VICE-PRESIDENT, BOOK
  OPERATIONS
Thomas A. Temple

VICE-PRESIDENT, PRODUCTION
  AND PURCHASING
Bacil Guiley

DIRECTOR, RESEARCH
Elizabeth O'Brien

Staff for this edition:
CLINICAL EDITOR: Paulette J. Strauch, RN
PHOTOGRAPHER: Paul A. Cohen
DESIGNER: Scott M. Stephens
COPY CHIEF: Jill Lasker
COPY EDITOR: Jo Lennon
EDITORIAL STAFF ASSISTANT: Katharine G. Morris
ART PRODUCTION MANAGER: Robert Perry
ARTISTS: Diane Fox, Donald G. Knauss, Sandra Sanders, Louise
  Stamper, Thom Staudenmayer, Joan Walsh, Robert Walsh
TYPOGRAPHY MANAGER: David C. Kosten
TYPOGRAPHY ASSISTANTS: Janice Haber, Ethel Halle, Diane Paluba,
  Nancy Wirs
PRODUCTION MANAGERS: Wilbur D. Davidson, Robert L. Dean, Jr.
COVER PHOTO: Paul A. Cohen

Clinical consultants for this edition:
Irving Huber, MD, *Assistant Professor, Department of Medicine and
  Surgery, Thomas Jefferson University Hospital, Philadelphia*
Kay L. Kilby, RN, *Emergency Trauma Coordinator, Wilmington (Del.)
  Medical Center*
Terri E. Weaver, RN, MSN, *Pulmonary Clinical Specialist, Hospital of the
  University of Pennsylvania, Philadelphia*

Staff for first edition:
BOOK EDITOR: Jean Robinson
CLINICAL EDITORS: Barbara McVan, RN, and
  Minnie Rose, RN, BSN, MEd
MARGINALIA EDITOR: Avery Rome
COPY EDITORS: Patricia Hamilton and Kathy Lorenc
RESEARCHER AND INDEXER: Vonda Heller
PRODUCTION MANAGER: Bernard Haas
PRODUCTION ASSISTANTS: David C. Kosten and Margie Tyson
DESIGNER: Maggie Arnott
ARTISTS: Bill Baker, Elizabeth Clark, Jack Crane, Owen Heinrich, Robert
  Jackson, Kim Milnazic, Robert Renn, and Sandra Sanders

Clinical consultants for first edition:
Betty L. Landon, RN, BA, *Associate Executive Director, Metropolitan
  Hospital, Springfield Division, Springfield, Pa.*
Romaine Hart, RN, *formerly Head Nurse, Cardio-Thoracic ICU,
  Hahnemann Hospital, Philadelphia*
Julieta D. Grosh, MD, FACS, *Surgical Director of Emergency
  Department, Temple University Hospital, Philadelphia*

Divider art by Fred Carbone
Photo on page 98 courtesy of Reeder, Sharon R., et al. *Maternity
  Nursing*, 15th ed. Philadelphia: J.B. Lippincott Co., 1976.

Library of Congress Cataloging in Publication Data

Main entry under title:

Giving emergency care competently.
  (New Nursing Skillbook)
  "Nursing83 books."
  Bibliography: p.
  Includes index.
  1. Emergency nursing. I. Series: [DNLM: 1. Critical care—Nursing texts.
  2. Emergencies—Nursing texts.   WY154 G539]
RT120.E4G58 1983   616'.025   83-16861
ISBN 0-916730-59-X

Contents

Contributors

Joy P. Clausen received her bachelor's and master's degrees in nursing from the University of Colorado, as well as her master's degree and doctorate in anthropology. Dr. Clausen is a professor in the College of Nursing at the University of Utah, Salt Lake City.

Jeanne Dupont is head nurse in the emergency department at the Massachusetts Eye and Ear Infirmary, Boston. She is a graduate of St. Elizabeth's School of Nursing in Boston and has given numerous lectures on the nursing care of eye emergencies.

Irving Feller is a clinical professor of surgery and director of the burn center at the University of Michigan. Dr. Feller is founder and director of the National Burn Information Exchange and founder and president of the Institute for Burn Medicine.

Margaret F. Fuhs is a pulmonary clinical specialist at the Hospital of the University of Pennsylvania in Philadelphia. She graduated from the Columbia University School of Nursing where she received her BSN. She received her MSN from the University of Pennsylvania. She is also working toward her doctorate in nursing at the Catholic University of America in Washington, D.C.

Peggy Eleanor Gordon received her bachelor's and master's degrees in nursing from the University of Virginia School of Nursing in Charlottesville, Virginia. She is a senior nurse at Friends' Hospital in Philadelphia.

Romaine Hart, one of the advisors on this book and author of the chapter on cardiac arrest, graduated from the Hahnemann Hospital School of Nursing in Philadelphia. She was formerly head nurse in the intensive care unit at Hahnemann Hospital.

Claudella Archambeault Jones is the educational administrator and director of the National Institute for Burn Medicine in Ann Arbor, Michigan. She received her education at the Mercy School of Nursing in Toledo, Ohio, and the University of Michigan in Ann Arbor.

Louise Juliani is an instructor at the University of Texas School of Nursing. She is a BSN graduate of the University of Wisconsin and has an MSN degree from Boston University.

Edward M. Lance is chief of the thoracic-cardiovascular section at the Jersey Shore Medical Center-Fitkin Hospital in Neptune, New Jersey. He is a graduate of Johns Hopkins University School of Medicine in Baltimore.

Betty L. Landon, one of the advisors on this book, is associate executive director at Metropolitan Hospital, Springfield Division, in Springfield, Pennsylvania. She is a graduate of Bellevue School of Nursing in New York City and earned her BA from the University of Redlands, Redlands, California.

Catherine Ciaverelli Manzi is a graduate of the Hahnemann Hospital School of Nursing, Philadelphia. She was formerly a nurse/researcher for *Nursing* magazine and is now a staff nurse in the intensive care unit of Frankford Hospital in Philadelphia.

Barbara F. McVan graduated from the Chestnut Hill School of Nursing in Philadelphia. She is one of the clinical editors of the Nursing Skillbook series, author of the chapter on anaphylactic shock, and one of the clinical directors in the Nursing Book Division.

Louise A. Milanese is a nurse consultant with Medeval, Philadelphia. She received her bachelor's degree in nursing at Holy Family College, Philadelphia.

Eileen Note received her bachelor's degree in nursing from Rutgers University College of Nursing and her master's from the University of Pennsylvania. She is a senior nurse at Friends' Hospital in Philadelphia.

Minnie Rose received her BSN from Indiana University in Bloomington and her master's degree in education from Temple University in Philadelphia. She was formerly assistant director of pharmacy in charge of the medication technician program at Temple, but is now one of the clinical editors of the Nursing Skillbook series and one of the clinical directors in the Nursing Book Division.

Hannelore Sweetwood is director of inservice education at Jersey Shore Medical Center, Neptune, New Jersey. Ms. Sweetwood graduated from Jersey City Medical Center School of Nursing and has a BS degree from Monmouth College in New Jersey.

Nancy Swift-Bandini graduated from the Frankford Hospital School of Nursing in Philadelphia and received her postgraduate education in neurosurgery at the National Hospital in London. Currently, she is a staff nurse in the neurologic intensive care unit at Hahnemann Hospital in Philadelphia.

Advisory Board

Foreword

If you've never saved a person's life—directly and single-handedly—then you have missed the greatest thrill possible in nursing. However, if you've tried but *failed,* you've experienced the greatest disappointment possible in nursing.

For that's the heart of nursing: saving lives. To do it, you must be trained correctly and be willing to treat whatever calamity that might appear, anytime day or night, and often without warning. It takes a special breed to do it well.

You are, or presumably would like to become, a member of that breed. It's not easy. It takes skills beyond those you learned in nursing school. It takes knowledge that can be recalled *stat*...when time won't permit research. For example, you need to know—instinctively—how to give cardiopulmonary resuscitation...how to deal with respiratory failure...when to summon a doctor immediately...which antidote to give...how to recognize impending shock...and how to carry out many, many other emergency procedures.

No matter where you work—in public health, hospital, industry, school, or wherever—these skills will serve you well. You *will* save lives, someday, if not every day.

Emergency care often involves public exposure, and this exposure adds another dimension to the situation. You'll meet patients of every age and social or economic level. You must be able to respond to them correctly—promptly. But you must be reassuring, too: positive, friendly, efficient. The public's reaction to their encounter with you can produce an opinion of your entire institution, an opinion that will stay in their minds for years.

In many emergency situations, you must also resign yourself to never knowing what eventually happens to the people you help. You'll see patients in precarious conditions. Then they'll become stabilized and leave. They may go home. Or they may go to surgery, or ICU, or someplace else. As soon as each one leaves, you'll go on with the job at hand. You won't have the luxury of time to sit and wonder what's happening to him.

Yes, good emergency nursing care takes finely honed

skills. That's why I was delighted to learn the publishers of *Nursing* magazine were creating this new book. It's truly an outstanding accomplishment. We nurses have a dearth of good, practical books about emergency care. And many are written solely for nurses who work in emergency departments.

This one encompasses both more and less than other books. It covers situations nurses might encounter outside the emergency department, as well as ones inside. Yet it covers only those emergencies that are truly life-threatening: emergencies when minutes or hours count.

I urge you to study this book carefully, again and again. Try to learn the procedures given by the many experts. Become fully prepared for the times when patients need you most. Work through the valuable Skillchecks to learn what you know and don't know.

If you haven't already experienced the thrill of directly saving a life, just wait. You will. And you'll be thankful that all of your preparation paid off.

You'll be a part of that special breed.

MARION Z. DOVER, RN
Member of the
Board of Directors
and Past President
of the Emergency Department
Nurses' Association (EDNA)

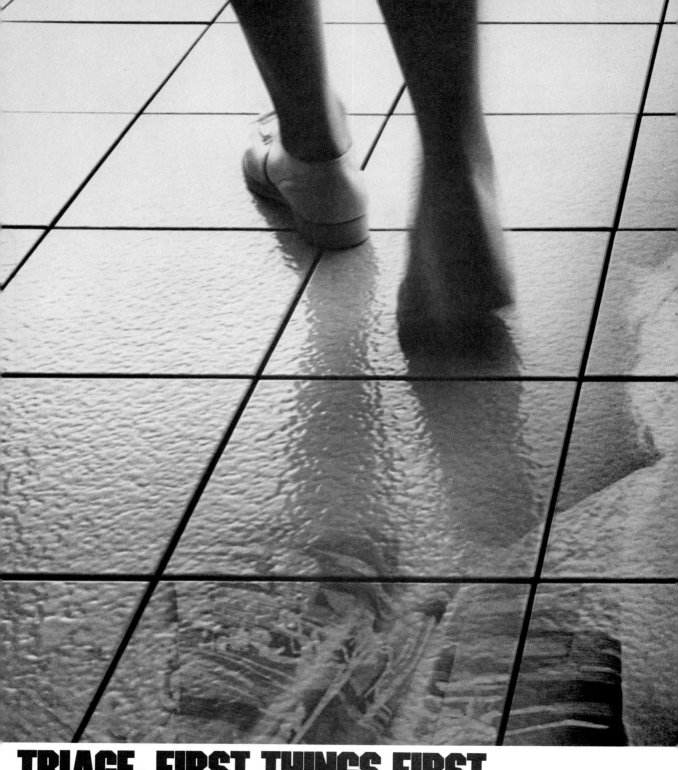

TRIAGE: FIRST THINGS FIRST

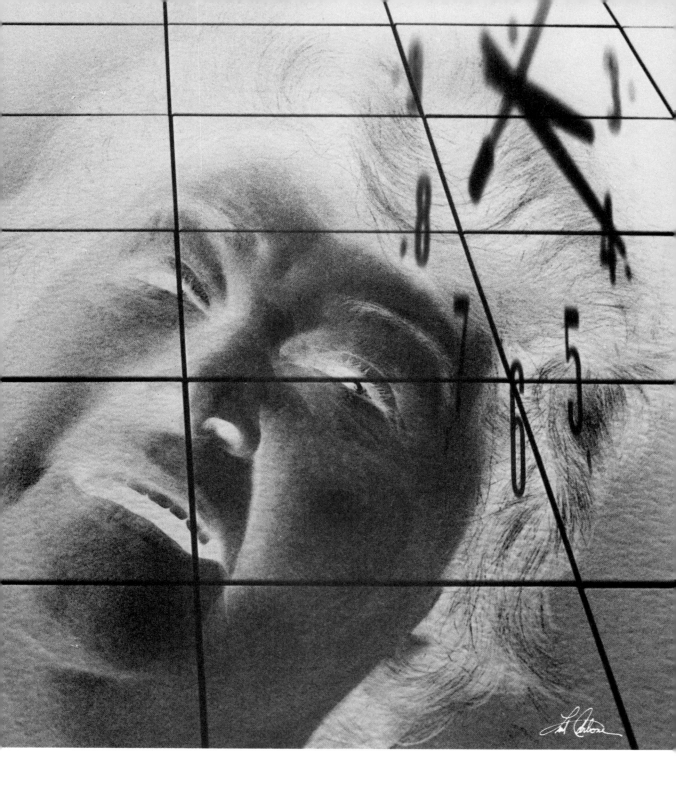

If your patient suffers cardiac arrest after being brought to the emergency department, what can you do to help distraught family members?

What can you do to establish priorities for a multiple trauma patient?

If your patient has an obstructed airway, what nursing actions can you take to open and clear it?

If a co-worker appears to have reached her stress limit, how can you help her?

How should you respond to a parent who shows no emotional reaction to his son's serious accident?

1

Triage
How to set priorities for patient care

BETTY L. LANDON, RN, BA

IMAGINE THAT YOU'RE a nurse in the emergency department of a big city hospital. Shortly after you arrive for work one morning, John Granger and his wife Sally are brought in with multiple injuries they suffered when their car was struck by a train. While you and the staff are busy treating them, another ambulance pulls up. This one has a couple and their five children, who were overcome by carbon monoxide from a faulty furnace.

Who'll assess the condition of these patients? Who'll decide which emergency comes first? What if *another* ambulance arrives within the next 10 minutes? How will you and the rest of the staff cope with the added stress?

Meet the triage nurse
That's where a triage nurse fits into the picture. Setting priorities for patient care is her responsibility. To do this, she examines a patient *immediately* upon his arrival and determines how serious his injury or illness is and what kind of care he needs.

In the case of the family overcome by carbon monoxide, one child was barely breathing and required immediate attention to save his life. The others had been sufficiently revived by ambulance attendants to wait for further treatment — although the triage nurse reexamined them every 15 minutes to make sure her assessment was still valid.

Not every emergency department has a triage nurse, of course. But every E.D. needs one. Triage seldom becomes just one nurse's responsibility because most hospitals assign the role on a rotating basis. Consider what could happen if one nurse had to take on this tremendous responsibility daily; in time, she might find it overwhelming. Role-changing in this case benefits her, as well as other staff members. Mimimizing stress in the emergency department — in whatever way possible — helps improve patient care.

The 90-second assessment

Let's talk more about the initial examination the triage nurse gives an incoming patient — and why it's so important. To illustrate, imagine a patient who's brought to the emergency department late one afternoon. He has a compound fracture of the right leg, which two of the nurses are attending to as the patient is transferred to another stretcher. One thing remains unnoticed, however. The patient also has an obstructed airway; as he was taken from the ambulance, he'd vomited and aspirated some of the vomitus.

Naturally, a patient could quickly die because of such an oversight — which points out the need for fast assessment. And by fast, I'm referring to the 90-second assessment explained on page 18. You can establish priorities for care using this guideline, because it covers the functions necessary to life: adequate, effective breathing and circulation.

If either of these are absent — or inadequate — you can start proper treatment immediately. And you won't waste precious seconds treating injuries or conditions that are less urgent.

Of course, the assessment checklist I've included in this chapter is only a guideline. You'll find more complete information on these emergency life-support measures in later chapters. But as a checklist, it shows what's included in the 90-second assessment — that all-important examination that every triage nurse should give. And I'm not referring to just emergency department triage; I'm talking about triage on every floor of the hospital — as well as triage in outpatient clinics, industrial settings, and institutions.

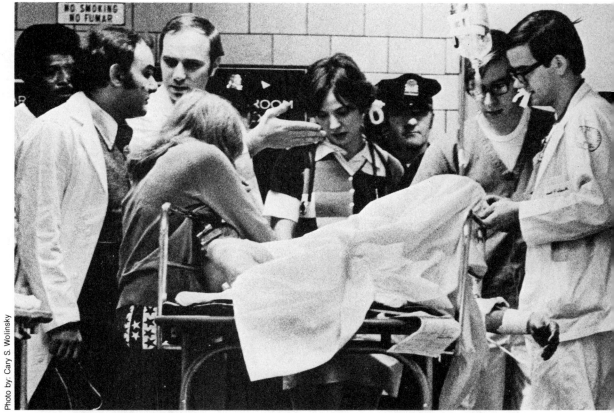

Knowing how to ask questions

But do more than observe the patient when you're setting priorities; *communicate* with him. Ask questions that'll get you a short medical history while you're doing the 90-second assessment.

Make them open-end questions, rather than questions that'll elicit just a yes or no answer. For example, *don't ask* a patient "Have you ever had a headache this bad before?" *Do ask* "When was the last time you had a headache this bad?"

You'll get more information about his injury or illness this way — and it'll probably be more accurate. Then you can record this information — along with your observations about his physical condition — on the form your hospital uses as a data collection sheet. (You'll find a sample of one of these forms, with an evaluation of Wilma Freelander, on page 19.)

The triage nurse as traffic cop

When a code is called, many staff members respond. Part of your job as triage nurse involves controlling the traffic in the emergency department. Make sure that extra personnel and family members leave so that only those people necessary to the patient's care remain in the room.

A IRWAY

Check the patient's airway for signs of obstruction: wheezing, stridor, or choking. If he makes a violent effort to sit up, let him do so. This may be a reflex action to establish an open airway.

PRIORITIES
* Position the patient on his back. Carefully straighten his arms and legs.

* Use the head-tilt–neck-lift or head-tilt–chin-lift maneuver to raise the tongue away from the back of the throat. In some cases this may be enough to start the patient breathing. *Caution:* When you suspect neck injury, don't use the head-tilt–neck-lift maneuver, but attempt to open the airway with a modified jaw-thrust.

* To treat airway obstruction: Insert oral or nasal airway, then suction patient. If patient is comatose, insert an endotracheal tube.

B REATHING

Check the patient's breathing to determine if his respirations are adequate. Look, listen, and feel for signs of breathing by placing your ear close to his mouth and nose to detect air movement. Watch his chest and abdomen to see if they rise and fall.

PRIORITIES:
* Auscultate breath sounds bilaterally.

* If the patient hasn't started breathing spontaneously after you've performed the head-tilt or jaw-thrust maneuver, ventilate him immediately using the mouth-to-mouth or mouth-to-nose technique shown on pages 34 and 35.
  Nursing tip: If the patient has a stoma from a tracheostomy, give mouth-to-stoma ventilations.
  You may also treat respiratory insufficiency with oxygen or positive-pressure ventilation.

C IRCULATION

Check the patient's circulation by feeling for a pulse in the carotid artery. If the neck has injuries, feel instead for a femoral pulse. If no pulse exists, the patient's circulation has stopped.

PRIORITIES:
* Perform closed-chest massage if circulation has stopped.

* Control external hemorrhage by applying direct pressure over the bleeding site.

* Control shock by administering I.V. fluids. Insert Foley catheter to measure output and assess fluid replacement. Measure vital signs and insert CVP line to monitor effectiveness of fluid replacement. Order arterial blood gas studies, complete blood count (CBC), blood urea nitrogen (BUN), glucose, and electrolytes to establish baseline values and monitor effectiveness of therapy.

The 90-second assessment
In an emergency, follow the ABCs of assessment to establish the priorities of your nursing care.

If you suspect neurologic damage, use the additional checklist in Chapter 12.

Coping with a bus strike

Let me tell you about 69-year-old Mrs. Freelander. Her case illustrates how much information a triage nurse can get by asking the right questions.

A neighbor who lived across the hall from Mrs. Freelander brought her into the E.D. after finding her slumped in a chair in her apartment. Mrs. Freelander moaned that she had such a severe headache that it had kept her from sleeping; in fact, she "couldn't tell for sure what day it was."

When the nurse asked her to describe the last time she'd had

DATA COLLECTION SHEET

Name: _Freelander, Wilma_   Age: _69_   Sex: _female_

1. What are the patient's symptoms? _Severe headache, nose bleeds X 2 in past week_

2. How long have these symptoms been present? _few days_
3. Has he/she been treated for them previously? Yes _____ No _X_
   If yes, in what way? _____
4. What is the patient's medical history? _hypertension_

5. Is he/she taking any medications? Yes _X_ No _____
   If yes, what? _was taking Aldomet until the supply ran out 10 days ago_
6. Does the patient have any other problems (for example, social or family) that may affect his illness? Describe: _Lack of transportation during bus strike_
7. List the patient's vital signs:
   Pulse _116_; Temperature _98°F_; Blood pressure _190/100_; Respirations _24_.
   Comments: _states blood pressure usually between 130 and 140_
8. Describe patient's state of consciousness (For example, is he/she alert, disoriented, responsive to painful stimuli, unresponsive?) Be sure to ask the person accompanying him what he's usually like. _Seems slightly confused as to time due to "severe headache"_

9. Describe the patient's general appearance (For example, is he cyanotic or jaundiced?) Don't forget to check his nail beds. _Skin color good nail beds pink_
10. Describe his behavior (Is he restless, anxious, hostile, depressed?) _Moaning, slightly restless, both hands holding head_

---

such a bad headache, Mrs. Freelander told her about one she'd had just a few days earlier. "It began right before a terrible nosebleed," she said. "My *second* nosebleed that week!"

As the nurse continued to question her, she found out other things: Mrs. Freelander was supposed to be taking methyldopa (Aldomet) for hypertension, but had discontinued it about 10 days earlier — when her supply ran out. Her reason: "I haven't been able to get to the drugstore, because of the bus strike," she explained. She didn't call her doctor about it, because she had been feeling fine without the medication.

It did matter, of course. Mrs. Freelander's headaches and nosebleeds were caused by her soaring blood pressure. It was 190/100, as you can see on the data collection sheet.

Getting a data base
Data collection sheets, like the sample above, should become part of the patient's permanent record. A well-documented sheet expedites the patient's care by giving the doctor essential information at a glance.

The challenge of children
Pediatric triage presents you with a unique challenge. Since young children and infants have immature organ systems, they respond unpredictably to bodily stresses. So ask the following important questions in your assessment:
• How old is the child?
• How long has he been ill?
• Does he *seem* very sick?
• Does he have trouble breathing?
• Does he have a fever?
• What condition made his parents bring him to the E.D.?
   Take the child's vital signs immediately. Examine him when he is awake and unclothed. Remember—the following conditions require immediate treatment:
• Difficulty breathing
• Fever, if the child is under 1 year old
• Ingestion of any toxic substance
• A sick or dehydrated appearance
• An alteration of consciousness.

Because the nurse knew how to ask questions, she was able to get the full story behind Mrs. Freelander's problem—and the doctor was able to make an accurate diagnosis. The triage nurse also had an opportunity to teach Mrs. Freelander why it's important to take her medicine as directed. And she notified the hospital's social service department, so they could help her get needed medicine for as long as the strike continued.

Maintaining good public relations
Setting priorities and collecting data aren't the only duties you'll have as a triage nurse. You must also keep everyone in the E.D. informed about the patients arriving there. You must:
• Advise the staff how many patients are still waiting for care, what condition they're in, and what kind of treatment they'll need.
• Inform members of the patient's family about his condition and comfort them. Remember, they usually can't accompany the patient into the treatment room and are probably anxious for news.
• Allay the fears of other patients, who have not yet been seen by a doctor, and reassure them that they haven't been forgotten. Sometimes, delays are caused by the sudden arrival of more urgent cases than theirs. If you inform waiting patients when this occurs, they're less likely to become upset.
   Nursing tip: Whenever you talk to a patient—or a patient's family—about his case, give him the privacy he deserves and don't discuss details in front of other people. Keep your voice low or, better yet, take the person you're talking to somewhere less crowded. Treat him as you would like to be treated, if you were in the same circumstances.

Remember these important points about triage:
1. Make your first priority a 90-second assessment of your patient's airway, breathing, and circulation.
2. Encourage the patient to communicate by asking open-ended questions.
3. Always fill out the data collection sheet as completely as possible. Note objective and subjective data.

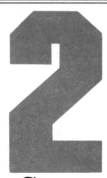

Stress
How you and others can cope

BETTY L. LANDON, RN, BA

THE TIME IS 7:05, one bitterly cold morning. You're working in the emergency department when a young woman rushes in with her 14-month-old son, whom she's wrapped in blankets because of the cold weather. She blurts out that he was hit by her babysitter for crying the night before — and now won't wake up. You remove the baby's blankets. You see at once that he's dead with multiple bruises and burns on his head and body.

Sympathy or anger?
What's your reaction to a case like this? Is it the same as either of these two nurses? One immediately felt sympathy for the bereaved mother; the other felt anger.

Which nurse was wrong in what she felt? The answer is, neither of them. You and the other staff members have a right to your feelings — same as everyone — and you need a chance to express them. That doesn't mean you should air your views in front of patients; although we've all seen cases in which this has happened. It means simply that a nonjudgmental environment must exist wherever you work, so you can express both positive and negative feelings without fear of censure.

Create a nonjudgmental environment

I want to help you create this kind of environment by what I say in this chapter. So I'll offer you some guidelines — guidelines that will enable you to interact successfully with everyone you deal with during an emergency. That includes more than just the patient; it also includes his family, other staff members, and sometimes the police and ambulance attendants. All of these people must cope with stress — many times on a daily basis — and all of them occasionally feel anger, hostility, and frustration.

Relate to the individual

Never forget you're dealing with individuals; don't expect everyone to respond exactly the same way. You've already seen this in the first case I mentioned, and now you'll see how it applies in the case of Walter Schaefer.

Mr. Schaefer's son was seriously injured when his car overturned on an icy road, but the first thing Mr. Schaefer asks about is the car. Doesn't he care about his son? Or is this just Mr. Schaefer's way of coping with unbearable stress?

Your intuition and experience tell you the latter answer is correct. Mr. Schaefer just can't deal with his son's condition at that moment. He needs more time and considerable support; his anguish is too great.

How should you respond in such a situation? Be patient, calm, and supportive. Never act judgmental. Don't say "Don't you care about your son?" Watch the person's face for clues about what he's really feeling. Listen to the *sound* of his voice; it may reveal more than the words he's saying.

If you're dealing with a patient or a member of his family, remember that you may be the first professional person to see him for that emergency. Your attitude toward him will make an impression and it may affect his behavior toward the rest of the staff. However, sometimes the patient reacts so poorly to stress that his normal support mechanisms fail and he becomes severely agitated, confused, or depressed. Chapter 17 explains how to deal with these psychiatric emergencies. Study it for details on what to do...and what not to do.

Know your limits

Not everyone can stand the same degree of stress on a day-to-day basis. Nor can everyone cope with stress indefinitely.

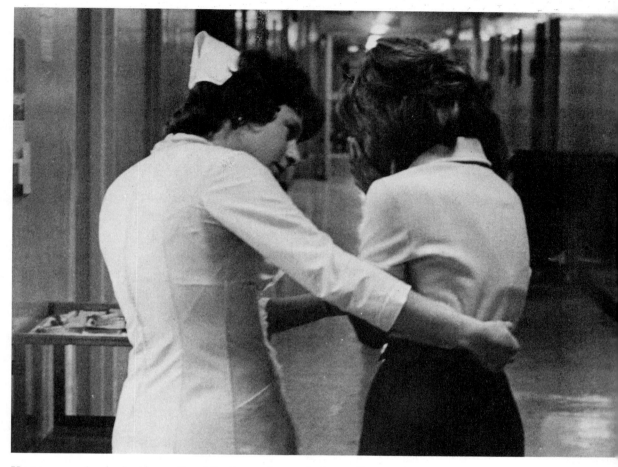

Know your physical and emotional limits, and — to the best of your ability — the limits of other staff members. If stress becomes more than you can manage successfully, find someone else to take your place — if possible. Be understanding when other staff members request relief. *Never permit any other staff member to criticize them for this.*

Show your appreciation
Help others cope with stress by showing how much you appreciate them. This is so basic that we tend to forget it. But a few words of appreciation go a long way, especially when you're tired and frustrated.

A private affair
A good triage nurse provides emotional support to the patient's family. Respect their need for privacy by using a quiet area for counseling. In a quiet environment you can provide information about the patient's condition and about the social services available in the hospital. Family members will be able to express their feelings more freely with the privacy they need.

Consider the case of an ambulance attendant I saw one night. He acted curt and unfriendly to everyone on the staff. But his attitude became understandable when we considered the unabated tension he'd been working under. In less than 6 hours, he'd brought three victims of automobile accidents, a severely burned child, and two patients in cardiac arrest to the E.D. He was suffering from stress; gruffness served as a way for him to cope with it. We helped him lessen that stress by telling him what a good job he was doing and how much we appreciated him.

Don't hesitate to say you understand how frustrating a person's job must be. This assures him that the tension he's feeling is valid. He's better able to cope with it, because he knows others understand what he's experiencing.

Be a good listener

Be a good listener when a patient or co-worker talks to you. To him, his problems deserve priority. But then, we all feel that way about our problems, so it's understandable.

Treat him as you would like to be treated. Give him your full attention. Don't let your eyes wander and don't keep glancing at your watch. Ask questions to clarify what you don't understand—or to help him focus on his problem. (For special hints on how to talk to patients or co-workers with problems, see Chapter 17.)

Try to arrange for group sessions in which you and other staff members can discuss your problems. But structure them in a way that will emphasize a positive look at situations. Make sure everyone agrees that the sessions stay nonjudgmental, so no one is censured for his feelings or attitude. Then truly listen to what each person says and try to understand him.

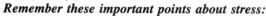

Remember these important points about stress:
1. Be calm and supportive when dealing with a patient or family member. Remember, your attitude may affect their behavior toward the rest of the staff.
2. Try to be aware of your stress level and the stress limits of other staff members.
3. Let others know how much you appreciate their efforts.
4. Be a good listener and never expect people to react the same way to a situation.

SKILLCHECK

1. You're doing triage in the emergency department of a big city hospital when Martin Rogers, a 48-year-old dress designer, is brought in suffering severe chest pains. As the doctor examines him, Mr. Rogers has a cardiac arrest and a Code is called to resuscitate him. Mrs. Rogers arrives from her home just minutes after all this has happened. She's understandably distraught. What can you do to help her?

2. The scene is the emergency department of a small coastline hospital, where Skip Brennan, a 20-year-old college student, is rushed after being hurt in a surfing accident. He's unconscious and appears to have head and neck injuries. The ambulance crew has placed him on a board and immobilized him with sandbags. Two of Skip's friends who have accompanied him to the hospital, refuse to leave his side. What do you do?

3. The emergency department has never seemed so busy. In the past hour, you've admitted 15 new patients. Only a few have injuries or conditions requiring immediate treatment, so the rest remain waiting to see a doctor. You've just told Mrs. Albert, who has a slightly sprained ankle, that she'll be next, when the ambulance arrives. You meet the paramedics at the door and learn that they're bringing in a family of six who were seriously injured in an automobile accident. What do you do next?

4. As the supervisor in a constantly busy emergency department, you know that stress can sometimes undermine a nurse's ability to cope. Nevertheless, you're surprised to find Rose Cerutti — one of your most experienced staff members — crying in the utility room. She sobs that she can't stand working the emergency department any longer and wants to quit. What do you do?

5. The day has been a tense one for everyone in the emergency department. More than one nurse has shown signs of stress, but none of them as acutely as Nellie Adams and Valerie Jameson. No matter what they do, these two nurses can't seem to communicate with each other effectively. Their rude exchanges make it impossible for them to work together cooperatively, and increase the overall tension in the E.D. Something has to be done immediately. Since you're the head nurse, what do you suggest?

6. Mary DeVito, a young RN, has been working in the emergency department for two months, under your supervision. One day, you learn from another nurse that Mary is angry and extremely frustrated about her minimal duties. Since she's had fewer duties than she expected for more than 2 weeks, she assumes that you're unhappy with her work or you would have given her additional responsibility. What can you say to help her in her new position?

7. James Gerhardt and his wife Julia arrive in the emergency department minutes after their 16-year-old daughter has died from injuries received in a car accident. They both hear the tragic news from the doctor, but only Mrs. Gerhardt breaks down and cries. Mr. Gerhardt doesn't seem to comprehend what has happened. When you try to offer your emotional support to him and Mrs. Gerhardt, he simply stares into space. What can you do?

(Answers on page 181)

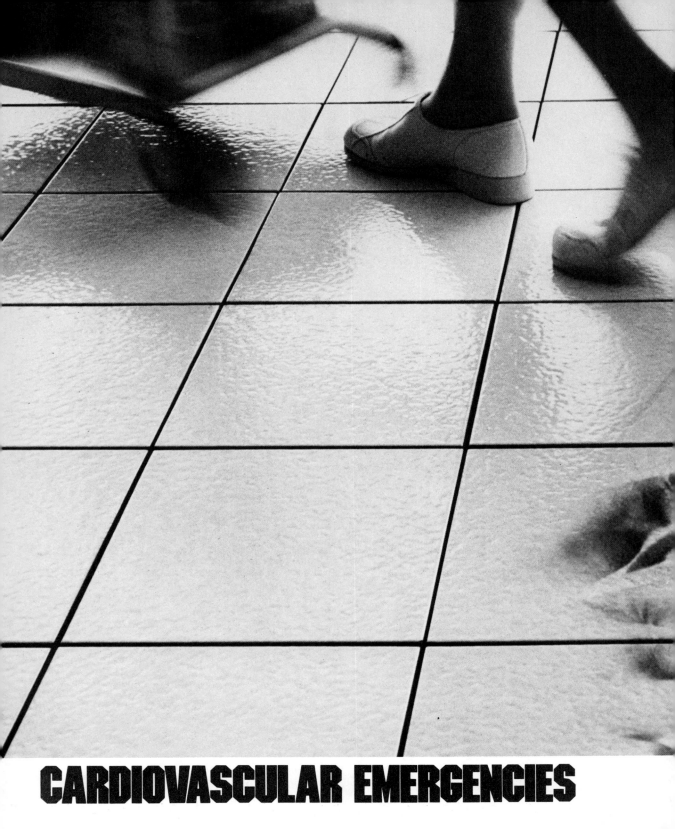

CARDIOVASCULAR EMERGENCIES

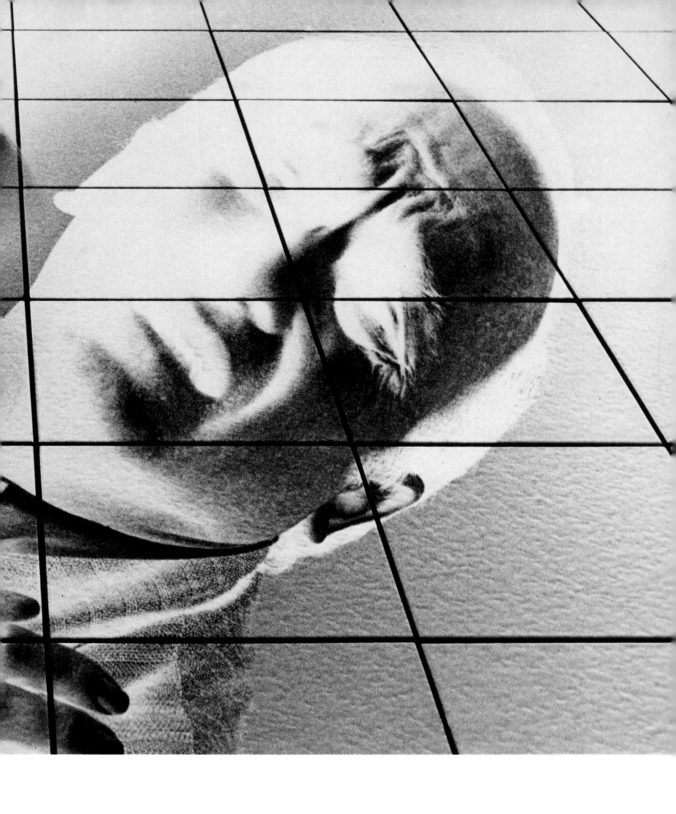

How do you quickly and accurately locate the best area of the chest for CPR?

If you're giving CPR to an adult and working alone, how many CPR chest compressions should you deliver per minute?

What areas of the body are most susceptible to frostbite?

If your patient has an open or penetrating abdominal wound, what is your first priority?

Can you differentiate between stable, unstable, and preinfarction angina?

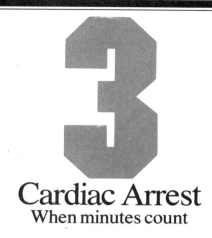

3

Cardiac Arrest
When minutes count

ROMAINE HART, RN

WHEN A MASSIVE midwinter blizzard closes roads and halts traffic one night, you and an LPN are the only nurses reporting for work on the surgical unit the next morning. Despite the extra workload, all seems to be going well for you and the remaining night-shift nurse for the first 2 hours. Then you stop to check 32-year-old Calvin Fox, who — up to then — had been recovering well from a nephrectomy. You find him lying unconscious on the floor near his bed. A quick examination tells you he's not breathing and has no palpable carotid pulse.

What now? Are you adequately trained to start cardiopulmonary resuscitation? What steps do you take while waiting for staff members to respond to your Code? When cardiac arrest occurs, you must work quickly to restore the patient's breathing and circulation. A brain deprived of oxygenated blood suffers irreversible damage in just 3 to 5 minutes.

As you know, you can successfully resuscitate a patient by working alone or with another staff member. But you both must be trained by a qualified CPR instructor to perform basic life-support techniques competently. In the following pages, I'm simply attempting to update your knowledge of CPR. Get your *full* training in the latest techniques from an instructor.

Opening the airway

You've just discovered an unconscious patient on the floor. Your first step, of course, is to check for signs of cardiac arrest so you'll know if you have to start CPR. Shake the patient's shoulders and call him by name to see if he responds. If he doesn't, quickly roll him over to a supine position and call for help.

Look, listen, and feel for signs of breathing. Place your ear close to his mouth and nose to detect air movement. Expose his chest and upper abdomen and watch for movement. No evidence of respiration means you must establish an open airway and begin artificial respiration.

When an unconscious patient lies in a supine position, his relaxed muscles allow his lower jaw to drop backward and permit his tongue to occlude his airway (see Figure 1). To relieve this obstruction quickly and easily, use the head-tilt maneuver shown in Figure 2. This raises the tongue away from the back of the throat, and in some cases may start the patient breathing.

Nursing tip: If your attempts to ventilate the patient show that you weren't able to open his airway with the head-tilt, try the jaw-thrust, as shown in Figure 3. To perform the jaw-thrust, place your fingers behind the angles of the patient's jaw and push it forward. Exert enough pressure to maintain the head-tilt.

Caution: Whenever you suspect neck injury in an unconscious patient, avoid using the head-tilt altogether and attempt to open his airway with a modified jaw-thrust. To do this, push the jaw forward, as shown in Figure 3, but don't hyperextend the neck or move the head to either side.

Ventilate the patient

If the patient still hasn't started breathing spontaneously, venti-late him immediately using the mouth-to-mouth or mouth-to-nose technique. To do the former, maintain his head-tilt position with your hands, as shown in Figure 4, and pinch his nostrils shut with your thumb and index finger. Take a deep breath. Now open your mouth wide and make a tight seal with your mouth. Blow air into his mouth, then remove your mouth from his so he can exhale. Try to start the patient breathing at this point by delivering 4 quick, full breaths with no time allowed between for full lung deflation.

If ventilation is impossible, reposition the head and attempt to ventilate again. If ventilation still isn't possible, give 4 back blows, followed by 4 abdominal thrusts. (See page 59 for details.)

Another way you can give artificial ventilation is mouth-to-nose. Use this method when the patient has a mouth injury or you're unable to form a tight seal over his mouth because he has no teeth.

If the patient has a stoma from a temporary tracheostomy, ventilate him in this way: Pinch his nostrils shut and seal his lips with your hand to prevent air leakage. Then put your mouth over his stoma and blow in air. Remove your mouth, so he can exhale. If he has a tracheostomy cannula in place, check for possible obstruction.

Assess circulation

Now check for a pulse in the carotid artery (see Figures 5 and 6). Use the external jugular vein, shown in Figure 5, as a reference point. If the neck has injuries, feel instead for a femoral pulse. If no pulse exists, the patient's circulation has stopped. Begin CPR immediately.

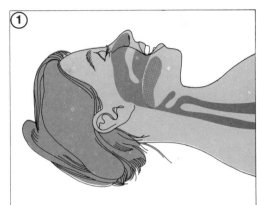

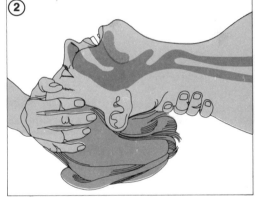

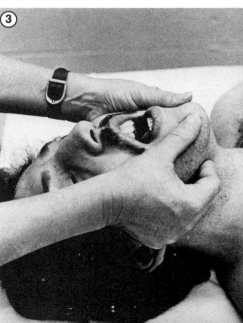

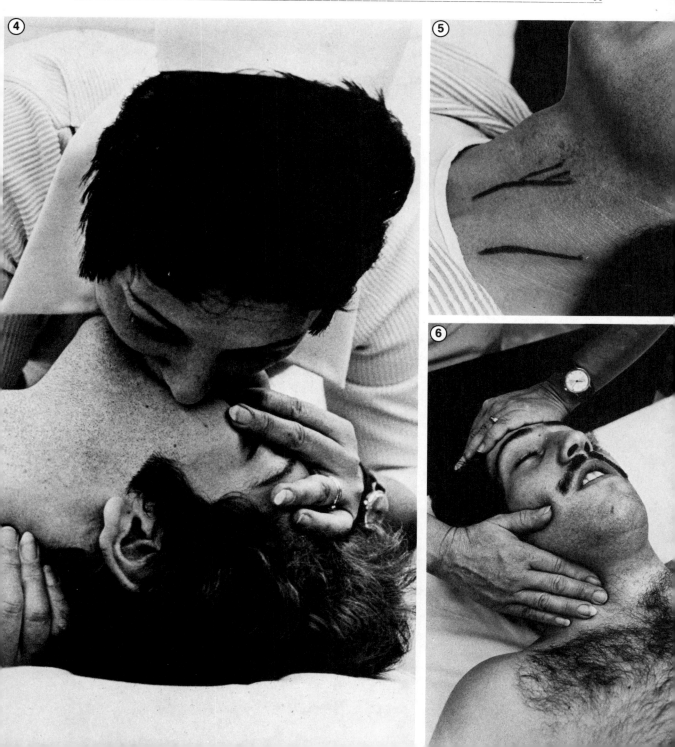

Restoring circulation

Before you proceed with CPR, check to be sure your patient's on a firm, flat surface. Then position yourself close to the patient's side with your knees apart. This position gives you a broad base of support.

Now, use the fingers of your hand that's closest to the patient's feet to find the correct hand position. Locate the lower margin of his rib cage and trace the margin to the notch where the ribs meet the sternum (see Figure 7). Next, place your middle finger on the notch (see Figure 8), and measure 1½″ to 2″—or approximately two finger-widths—*up from this point* (see Figure 9). You'll give chest compressions in this area.

Caution: If your hands are positioned incorrectly, you may fracture your patient's ribs and cause further problems, such as a liver laceration.

Next, place the hand you used to locate the notch over the heel of your other hand. Interlock or extend your fingers to keep them off the patient's ribs and to maintain vertical pressure through the heel of the hand touching the sterum (see Figure 10). Bring your shoulder directly over the patient's sternum, keeping your arms absolutely straight (Figure 11). Establish a position in which your shoulders are at a right angle to the patient's chest, then begin downward

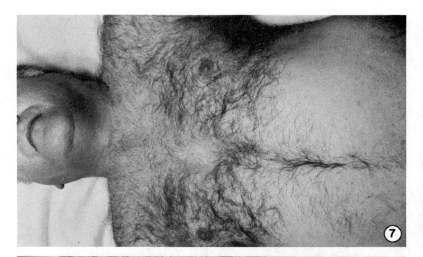

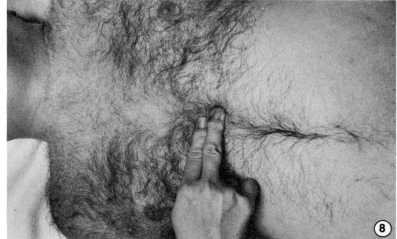

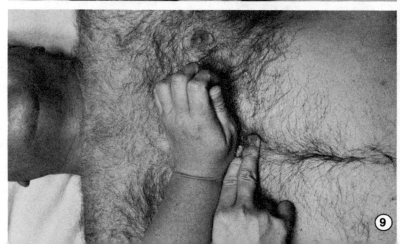

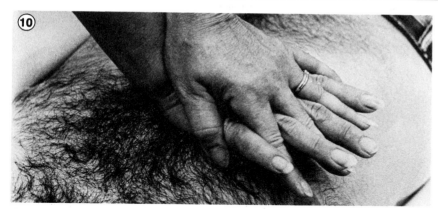

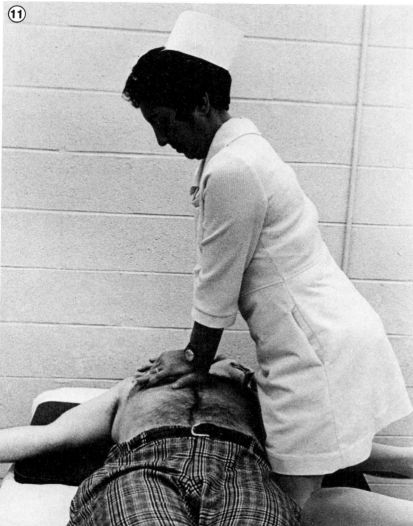

compressions, depressing the sternum 1½" to 2". This movement squeezes the heart between the sternum and the vertebral column, forcing blood from the chambers.

After each compression, release the pressure, allowing the sternum to return to its normal position. This action permits the heart's chambers to refill. Compression and relaxation time must be of equal duration.

Perform this compression-release sequence in a regular, uninterrupted rhythm: 80 per minute, if you are working alone; 60 per minute, if two nurses are working as a team.

Obviously, to be effective, you must give the patient artificial respiration at the same time you're applying external chest compressions (refer back to Figure 4). If you're alone, accomplish this by giving the patient 2 quick lung inflations after each 15 chest compressions. Deliver these in rapid succession (within a period of 5 seconds), not allowing for full lung exhalation between breaths.

Watch the patient's chest while you're working to see if your ventilations are effective. After the first minute of chest compressions, check his carotid pulse. An adequate compression should produce a palpable carotid pulse, unless, of course, the patient has already expired.

Working as a team

If another nurse can help you
give CPR, one of you should
inflate the patient's lungs while
the other applies external chest
compressions. You can position
yourself as shown in Figure 12,
but if CPR must continue for
an extended period of time, you'll
be better off working on opposite sides of the patient. This will
permit you to shift tasks without
interrupting the compression-
relaxation and ventilation cycle
necessary for effective cardiopulmonary resuscitation.

Work as a team, remembering
that 1 lung inflation must be
given after every 5 chest compressions. Deliver the lung inflations quickly, so there's no
pause in compressions. To be
effective, the compression-
release sequence for team CPR
must be 60 per minute, with
1 lung inflation interposed between every 5 compressions.

If the person giving chest
compressions tires and needs to
switch positions, she notifies
her helper by saying (in rhythm),
"Change one-thousand, two-
one thousand, three-one thousand, four-one thousand, five-
one thousand." Then, the helper
giving lung inflations delivers
one breath and moves into position for chest compressions.
Now the person giving chest
compressions completes the
compression sequence, moves
next to the patient's head and
checks his carotid pulse for
5 seconds, *but no longer.* If no
carotid pulse is felt, she delivers
a breath and tells the helper
giving chest compressions,
"continue CPR." But if she feels
a carotid pulse she'll say,
"there's a pulse" and continue to
give artificial respiration.

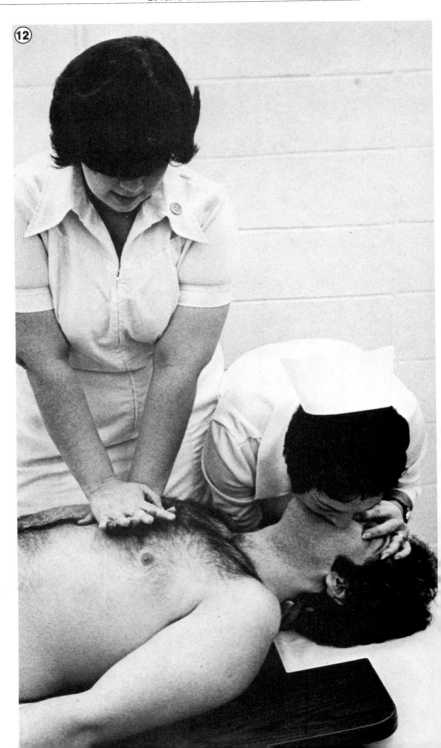

⑫

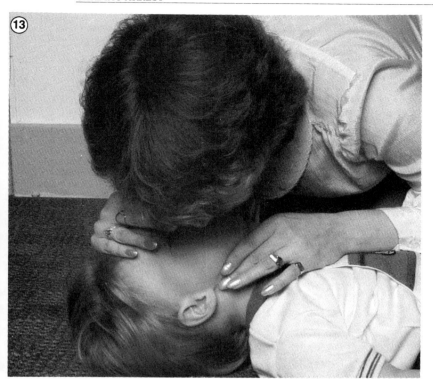

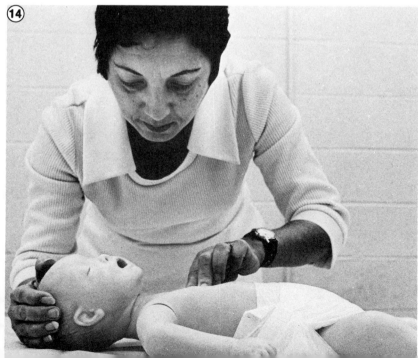

CPR for children

When you give CPR to a child or infant, remember that the basic procedure is the same—with some modifications. For example, don't hyperextend a child's or infant's neck as much as you would an adult's. If you did, you could damage his spine and cause serious neurologic damage. As shown in Figure 13, ventilate a very young patient by sealing both his mouth and nose with your mouth. Give *small* breaths to inflate the lungs, interposing 1 lung inflation between every 5 chest compressions. The compression rate should be 80 per minute for a child, or 100 per minute for an infant.

As you can see from Figure 14, giving chest compressions to an infant is quite different from giving chest compressions to an adult. For infants, use only the tips of your index and middle fingers to compress the midsternum between the nipples ½″ to 1″. For children, use only the heel of one hand to compress the sternum 1″ to 1½″. More forceful chest compressions could lacerate the patient's liver. If you have difficulty with ventilations, check for airway obstruction, as explained in Chapter 6.

A very young patient can easily develop gastric distention when he's given artificial ventilation. If distention seems marked, relieve it by applying gentle pressure over the upper epigastric region. Turn the patient on his side so he doesn't aspirate vomitus. Clear his airway before continuing CPR.

Remember these important points when caring for a patient in cardiac arrest:

1. No evidence of respiration means you must establish an open airway and begin artificial respiration immediately.

2. Use three methods to open an airway: the preferred head-tilt–chin-lift, the head-tilt–neck-lift, or the jaw-thrust without head-tilt.

3. To open an infant's airway, support his back with the hand closest to his feet or a rolled towel, and gently tilt his head back.

4. To relieve marked gastric distention in a child during artificial ventilation, apply gentle pressure over the upper epigastric region.

5. Ventilate a laryngectomee using the mouth to stoma method.

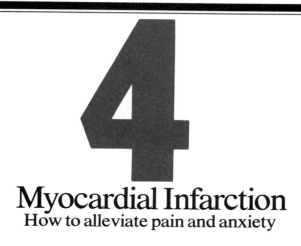

Myocardial Infarction
How to alleviate pain and anxiety

CATHERINE CIAVERELLI MANZI, RN

"POSSIBLE MI!" For you, these words mean emergency. When you learn that a patient with a possible myocardial infarction is coming to the emergency department, you've got to be ready to give him what he needs: emotional support and a quick, accurate assessment.

Do you know how to supply these needs? In many cases, a nurse is the first professional to see the patient in a hospital. Are you adequately informed, so you know what steps to take immediately with each patient — and what problems you might encounter? For example, do you know how to connect the patient to the monitor or EKG machine properly? Do you know how to interpret a rhythm strip? Do you know what to do for a life-threatening arrhythmia if the patient develops one? What must you ask the patient to help the doctor make an accurate diagnosis? Using a case history to illustrate, I'll answer these questions for you in this chapter.

Introducing Otto Frankenfeld
You've been alerted that a patient with a possible MI will be coming to the E.D. And soon after, ambulance attendants wheel in 56-year-old Otto Frankenfeld. He looks pale, is

diaphoretic and seems extremely upset. He gasps that his chest feels like someone is sitting on it, and the pain, which is severe, goes down his left arm.

His distressed wife tells you that he started having episodes of severe chest pain earlier that evening, while they were attending a concert. Each episode lasted from 5 to 10 minutes. "When he started having the third one, I got someone to call an ambulance," she whispers frantically. "Is he having a heart attack? Is he going to... die?"

What to do first
Naturally, you can't be sure Mr. Frankenfeld has an acute MI at first. As you can see on the opposite page, many other things cause similar chest pain. The doctor must first assess Mr. Frankenfeld's overall condition to get an accurate diagnosis. But you can help Mr. Frankenfeld, and aid the doctor in his examination, by following the priorities discussed below.

As you follow these priorities, remember that you can't always do them in order. Many times, your first nursing action is in response to the patient's most pressing need. For example, you might treat his pain first—if it's extremely severe—because continued pain can lead to shock or extension of the MI. Set your priorities according to the patient's needs or perform them simultaneously with the help of other staff members.

Introduce yourself to the patient and start taking his history as soon as possible. At the same time, *use your eyes* and watch the patient closely. Observe his general appearance, his facial expressions, his skin color, and the tracings on his monitor.

Ask him about his chest discomfort. Be patient as you do this, and try not to ask leading questions. For example, don't say "Does your discomfort feel like someone is sitting on your chest, or is it a squeezing or stabbing sensation?" Instead, ask him to describe exactly how the discomfort feels. Ask him when it started, how long each episode lasted, and how many times he's had them. Let him show you exactly where he feels the discomfort.

Nursing tip: If your patient's gripping his chest, note the location of his hands. Consider hand position a clue to pain location.

What was he doing *before* the pain started? Has he ever had

HOW VARIOUS KINDS OF CHEST PAIN DIFFER				
	ONSET AND DURATION	LOCATION AND RADIATION	QUALITY AND INTENSITY	SIGNS AND SYMPTOMS	PRECIPITATING FACTORS
Myocardial infarction	Sudden onset: pain ½ to 2 hr; residual soreness, 1 to 3 days	Substernal, midline, or anterior chest pain; radiation down one or both arms to jaw, neck, or back	Severe pressure, deep sensation: "crushing," "stabbing," "viselike"	Apprehension, nausea, dyspnea, diaphoresis, increased pulse, decreased blood pressure, gallop heart sound	Occurrence at rest or with exertion, physical or emotional
Angina (stable, unstable, and preinfarction)	Stable: gradual onset; predictable pattern less than 15 min and not more than 30 min Unstable: gradual onset; may occur or reoccur spontaneously; not relieved by nitroglycerin or rest Preinfarction: sudden onset; lasts longer than stable or unstable angina	Substernal or anterior chest pain, not sharply localized; radiation to back, neck, arms, jaw, even upper abdomen or fingers	Mild to moderate pressure, uniform pattern of attacks; deep sensation, tightness, squeezing, "viselike"	Dyspnea, diaphoresis, nausea, desire to void, belching, apprehension; elevated blood pressure and increased heart rate immediately before or occuring at onset	Exertion, including sexual intercourse; stress; eating; micturition or defecation; cold or hot, humid weather
Pericarditis	Sudden onset; continuous pain lasting for days; residual soreness	Substernal pain to left of midline; radiation to back or subclavicular area	Mild ache to severe pain, deep or superficial: "stabbing," "knifelike"	Precordial friction rub; increased pain with movement, inspiration, laughing, coughing, left side position; decreased pain with sitting or leaning forward	Myocardial infarction or upper respiratory infection; no relation to effort
Pleuropulmonary	Gradual or sudden onset; continuous pain for hours	Pain over lung fields to side and back; radiation to anterior chest, shoulder, or neck	Deep sharp ache, "knifelike," "shooting," "crushing"	Pleural rub, fever, dyspnea; increasing pain with coughing, inspiration, and movement; decreased pain with sitting	Pneumonia or other respiratory infection
Esophagealgastric	Gradual or sudden onset; continuous or intermittent pain	Substernal, midline, or anterior chest pain; radiation to upper abdomen, back, or shoulder	Squeezing pain, heartburn	Dysphagia, belching, vomiting, diaphoresis, reflux esophagitis, decreased pain with sitting or standing	Ingestion of alcohol or spicy foods, history of gastrointestinal problems
Musculoskeletal	Gradual or sudden onset; continuous or intermittent pain	To right or left of midline	Soreness	Increased pain with movement	History of previous neck and arm injury

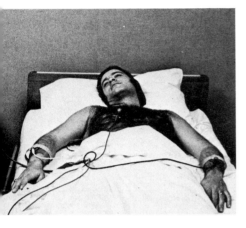

EKG tips
Here are some EKG pointers you
can use in a hospital, doctor's
office, or outpatient department.
1. Find out if the patient has
ever had an EKG before. Explain
the procedure carefully (some
patients think you're going to
electrocute them!), and assure
him that it's painless.
2. Take a patient history. Ask if
he's taking any drugs, if he has a
pacemaker, and so on. Record
the information.
3. Tell the patient to relax, lie
flat, and breathe normally. Older
patients with orthopnea may
need more than one pillow.
4. Protect the patient's privacy.
Draping a towel over a woman's
chest will make her feel more
comfortable.
5. Observe the patient during
the test. Correlate any movement
or activity with the tracing. If
you spot an arrhythmia, get a
good tracing as you watch the
patient closely for corresponding
symptoms.

pain like this before? If he has, how is it similar? Is there any
way that it's different? Does he take any medication for chest
pain or discomfort? Ask what the medication is.

Important nursing tip: If the patient has taken a nitroglycerin
tablet for angina, be sure to ask him if he felt a burning sensation when he placed it under his tongue. Absence of this
sensation indicates that the tablet has lost its potency and the
supply needs to be replaced.

Connect the patient to a cardiac monitor and obtain a rhythm
strip. Make sure the monitor is operating properly. Is the tracing clear? Can you distinguish the wave patterns easily? Set
your rate parameters. Adjust the gain or size dial of the monitor, if necessary. Make sure the alarm or audio signal works.
If you don't receive a clear tracing, check the electrode wires
to see if you have a tight connection. Try changing the position
of the electrodes on the patient or test the cable and wires with
a tester, if one is available.

Some E.D.'s don't have individual monitors, however. If
not, connect the patient to a 3- or 5-lead EKG machine and
get a rhythm strip every 15 to 30 minutes. Otherwise, take the
EKG after your patient's connected to the monitor.

Now draw a blood sample for complete blood count (CBC),
electrolytes, and arterial blood gases. Be sure cardiac enzymes, as well as isoenzymes, are tested; this is especially
important when the patient has a possible MI. Start an I.V.
with 5% dextrose in water.

Observe and evaluate
Keep observing the patient and evaluating his pain as to its
character, duration, location, and frequency. Try to assess his
anxiety level. Remember, anxiety may increase pain by speed-
ing up the heart rate and elevating blood pressure. These two
conditions increase myocardial oxygen consumption.

Most MI patients need medication to provide constant pain
relief with controlled blood level and to help reduce myocardial oxygen consumption. The doctor will probably order lidocaine and nitroglycerin I.V. (Nitrostat or Tridil). Lidocaine
helps prevent life-threatening arrhythmias, while nitroglycerin
I.V. relieves signs and symptoms of angina pectoris unrelieved
by nitroglycerin tablets or beta blockers. Before you give any
drug, determine if the patient has any allergy to it. Watch your
patient closely for side effects associated with these drugs.

Have oxygen on hand, and be ready to administer it by nasal cannula at 6 to 8 liters per minute—or as the doctor orders. Be sure to check if the patient has a history of respiratory problems. If he does, the doctor will probably order oxygen to be administered at 1 to 2 liters per minute to reduce the risk of respiratory arrest.

Check and record the patient's vital signs, so you'll have a baseline for comparison later. Listen to his lungs for rales and to his heart for a gallop rhythm, which could indicate left ventricular failure or dysfunction. Are his neck veins distended when he's at a 45° angle? If so, note this on your record. Neck-vein distention reflects the venous pressure of the right atrium.

The doctor will probably want to draw an arterial blood sample to measure its oxygen content. Explain this test to the patient as you set up the equipment. Then when the sample is taken, hold pressure on the puncture site for at least 10 minutes. Make sure no air bubbles exist in the syringe. Place the syringe on ice immediately. Label the sample with the patient's name, date, and time. *Important:* Has the patient received oxygen for at least 30 minutes prior to that time? If so, record the O_2 flow liters per minute on the lab slip.

Give the patient emotional support and reassurance. I can't stress this enough. Remember, when a patient's having an MI—or thinks he's having an MI—he's extremely anxious and afraid of dying. He sees the unfamiliar faces of nurses, doctors, and technicians around him. The equipment and procedures in the E.D. seem strange and frightening. And he knows his family is probably standing by, worrying.

So do what you can to alleviate his anxiety. Speak to him slowly and calmly. Encourage him to express his feelings to you...and then listen. Explain what to expect, but don't give him false reassurances. Don't say "Everything will be all right." He knows everything may *not* be all right. Be understanding. Many times an anxious patient needs repeated explanations of what is happening to him, as well as repeated reassurances that you're trying to help him. Keep his family informed about his condition, and tell him you've done so.

Getting a diagnosis
Let's consider the importance of laboratory findings in making a diagnosis: for example, cardiac enzyme levels. As you

NORMAL CARDIAC SERUM ENZYME LEVELS				
CARDIAC ENZYME	NORMAL SERUM LEVELS	ELEVATION (POST MI)		
		ONSET	PEAK	END
Creatine phosphokinase CPK	Male: 23 to 99 units/liter Female: 15 to 57 units/liter	Within 1 day	Within 1 day	1 to 2 days
Serum glutamic-oxaloacetic transaminase SGOT	8 to 20 units/liter	1 day	1 to 2 days	4 to 6 days
Lactic dehydrogenase LDH	48 to 115 units/liter	2 days	2 to 5 days	4 to 6 days
Alpha-hydroxybutyric dehydrogenase HBD	114 to 290 units/ml	2 days	3 days	14 days
Serum glutamic-pyruvic transaminase SGPT	Male: 10 to 32 units/liter Female: 9 to 24 units/liter	SGPT levels usually remain near normal except in patients with liver disease.		

Here's a handy chart showing you at a glance the normal cardiac serum enzyme levels. You can also see when elevations will likely occur postinfarction.

know, enzymes are naturally occurring compounds found in all tissues. Each tissue has its own enzymes, though some enzymes are found in more than one kind of tissue. When tissue gets damaged—as in a myocardial infarction—the enzymes escape into the bloodstream. Thus an elevated cardiac enzyme level in a patient's blood sample suggests myocardial infarction.

Which enzymes are measured to diagnose an MI? They are creatine phosphokinase (CPK), serum glutamic-oxaloacetic transaminase (SGOT), and lactic dehydrogenase (LDH). You should check them on admission, then once a day for the next 3 days.

If Mr. Frankenfeld has suffered a myocardial infarction, you'd expect his CPK level to rise within 1 day after his attack, his SGOT level to rise in 1 day, and his LDH level to rise within 2 days.

Sometimes the cardiac enzyme levels, when first measured, are normal in a patient with MI. This can happen when he gets to the E.D. quickly; that's one of the reasons you must ask when his chest discomfort started—it can make a difference. Remember, even though enzyme levels can be used to diagnose

MI, they're not relied on exclusively. A doctor also depends on EKG findings and information from the patient's case history.

Nursing tip: Since CPK levels rise with muscle injury, try to obtain the blood sample for this test *before* giving an I.M. injection. However, some hospital laboratories can fraction out the CPK or LDH enzymes and tell which percentage of the enzyme is coming from skeletal muscle tissue and which percentage from myocardial tissue.

Now let's get back to the EKG that you took on Mr. Frankenfeld. What do you look for that will tell you whether or not he's suffered ischemia or injury to his myocardium? Look for changes in the S-T segment, such as elevation and/or depression. Myocardial infarction can occur in the septum or in the anterior, posterior, inferior, or lateral walls of the myocardium. Specific leads on the EKG show the condition of those areas.

Usually, you'll see elevation in leads representing the infarcted area and S-T segment depression in leads representing an uninjured area. In an MI, S-T segment elevation usually indicates myocardial injury with T wave inversion. However, the doctor won't arrive at a final diagnosis until he sees pathological Q waves with the above. A pathological Q wave of 1 mm or greater in depth indicates necrosis and appears within 48 hours after an infarction. (Naturally, you'll only see this Q wave and the above changes in leads representing the infarcted area.)

Of course, the absence of any of these EKG findings on admission doesn't necessarily rule out a myocardial infarction. These changes may be delayed for hours or even days; that's why the doctor orders serial tracings to follow the heart's electrical activity for 3 or more days.

Mr. Frankenfeld's EKG findings suggested an acute inferior wall infarction. To learn more about what I've told you here, read the *Nursing Skillbook,* READING EKGs CORRECTLY.

Watch out for arrhythmias

Mr. Frankenfeld could develop a life-threatening arrhythmia or go into cardiac arrest at any time—because of myocardial ischemia, hypotension, impaired pulmonary ventilation, or drug therapy. The most common complication after acute MI is a ventricular arrhythmia, though other arrhythmias can occur, depending on the infarction's location.

Watch closely for premature ventricular contractions (PVCs), which may precede ventricular tachycardia. If they're back-to-back, or occurring at a rate of five or more per minute, treat them with the emergency drugs the doctor has standing orders for. Usually, you'll administer a lidocaine bolus of 50 to 100 mg, then start a lidocaine drip (2 g in 500 cc of 5% dextrose in water) to run at a rate of 1 to 4 mg per minute. The maintenance dosage of lidocaine depends on the patient's response to the drug.

Nursing tip: Always use microdrip tubing when administering lidocaine to avoid giving an accidental drug overdose.

If ventricular tachycardia or cardiac arrest occurs, start cardiopulmonary resuscitation (see Chapter 3) and give the appropriate emergency drugs.

Remember, watching the patient's EKG monitor can't substitute for personally checking his condition. Record his vital signs every 10 to 15 minutes until he's stable enough to be transferred to the CCU or ICU. Ask him how he feels, touch his skin, note his general appearance, and record the quality and frequency of his respirations. Remind him to tell you at once if he has further chest pains or discomfort after he receives pain medication. (Increased chest pain may mean an extension of his MI.) Be prepared for any life-threatening changes in your patient's condition by keeping emergency equipment and drugs on hand.

Remember these important points when caring for a patient with a possible myocardial infarction:
1. Ask your patient objective and subjective questions about his chest discomfort. An accurate patient history is the most important tool in an emergency department diagnosis of a myocardial infarction.
2. Always evaluate chest pain onset, duration, radiation, and character, as well as associated signs and symptoms.
3. Usually, you'll connect your patient to a cardiac monitor before taking a 3- or 5-lead EKG.
4. Look for elevation and/or depression in the S-T segment of the patient's EKG. If present, suspect injury to the myocardium.
5. Be alert for life-threatening arrhythmias. If they occur, follow the doctor's standing orders.

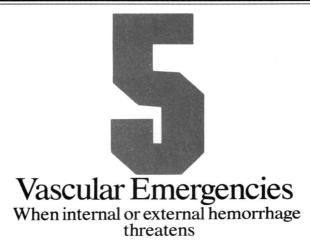

Vascular Emergencies
When internal or external hemorrhage threatens

MINNIE ROSE, RN, BSN, MEd

VASCULAR EMERGENCIES POSE many nursing problems. If you aren't prepared to act properly and efficiently, the patient can bleed to death in a matter of minutes. Do you know how to recognize vascular obstruction? Can you initiate the appropriate treatment for internal as well as external hemorrhages? Are you familiar with the symptoms of an embolus, of venous thrombosis, or of an aneurysm?

You'll find the answers to these questions and what to do about these conditions in this chapter. Remember — regardless of the cause, a vascular emergency threatens the patient's life until either the cause or the patient is defeated.

Fighting a hemorrhage
Let's suppose Louise Scott is admitted to the emergency department with hemorrhage from a laceration of her left wrist. You summon help and then begin assessing and caring for her injury. Although massive external hemorrhage like Ms. Scott's can disturb everyone involved, it seldom threatens a patient's life as much as internal hemorrhage.

However, when hemorrhage of any kind causes severe loss of circulating blood volume, the patient will die unless the

How to control a hemorrhage
The drawings on the opposite
page show you where to apply
pressure to control hemorrhage in
any part of the body. You should
be completely familiar with these
pressure points, so that you are
prepared for a vascular
emergency.
1. For a wound of the scalp or
temple, compress the temporal
artery.
2. For a wound of the lower face
(below the eyes), apply pressure
to the facial artery along the lower
border of the mandible.
3. For a neck wound, compress
the wound site. Do not compress
the carotid artery, as this could
cause stroke.
4. For a shoulder wound or
hemorrhage of the upper arm,
compress the subclavian artery
against the clavicle.
5. For a wound of the lower part of
the upper arm or of the elbow,
press the brachial artery against
the humerus.
6. For foot wounds, compress the
entire network of arteries in the
ankle.
7. For a wound of the lower arm,
press the ulnar and radial arteries
at the antecubital fossa.
8. For hand wounds, press the
ulnar and radial arteries at the
wrist.
9. For thigh wounds, apply great
pressure to the femoral artery
against the femur.
10. For wounds of the lower leg,
apply pressure to the popliteal
artery, behind the knee.

blood volume can be restored quickly. The body's own protective mechanisms initiate a temporary vasoconstriction to maintain blood pressure, and the blood starts clotting at the injury site. But in severe cases these measures will be inadequate. The loss of blood volume will cause blood pressure to fall, and shock symptoms will begin. Arterial hemorrhage is usually more serious than venous hemorrhage because each heartbeat forces the blood to spurt out under maximum pressure. You can determine the hemorrhage's severity by the type, the number, and the location of the vessels involved.

While you're waiting for the doctor to arrive, apply direct pressure to Ms. Scott's wound with a sterile gauze pad and elevate her arm. (If, under other circumstances, you suspected she also had a fracture, you wouldn't elevate her arm; that could cause further damage.) Avoid using a tourniquet to control bleeding since it would risk gangrene. Use tourniquets only when you can't control a life-threatening hemorrhage by other means.

Check Ms. Scott's vital signs; then test her for possible damage to the nerves and the tendon in her arm. Since her cut was superficial, Ms. Scott escaped neurological and tendon damage to her wrist and needed only sutures to close her wound.

The "two-sided" patient
Ms. Scott's injury was one of the less severe vascular emergencies you'll see in an emergency department. To help a patient like her, you must recognize relevant symptoms, initiate appropriate treatment, and obtain baseline data.

For a patient with a vascular emergency that requires more complex treatment, follow these guidelines:

• Does he have adequate ventilation? Remove any airway obstruction and use a pharyngeal airway, oxygen, or suctioning as needed.

• Did you take vital signs on both sides of the body? Think of the patient as two-sided: Palpate paired pulses and take blood pressures in both arms. If the blood pressure in one arm is lower than in the other, suspect an obstruction or vascular deficit.

• Is he free from pain when he should be experiencing some? This could indicate sensory damage.

• Has his normal skin color changed? In Caucasian patients,

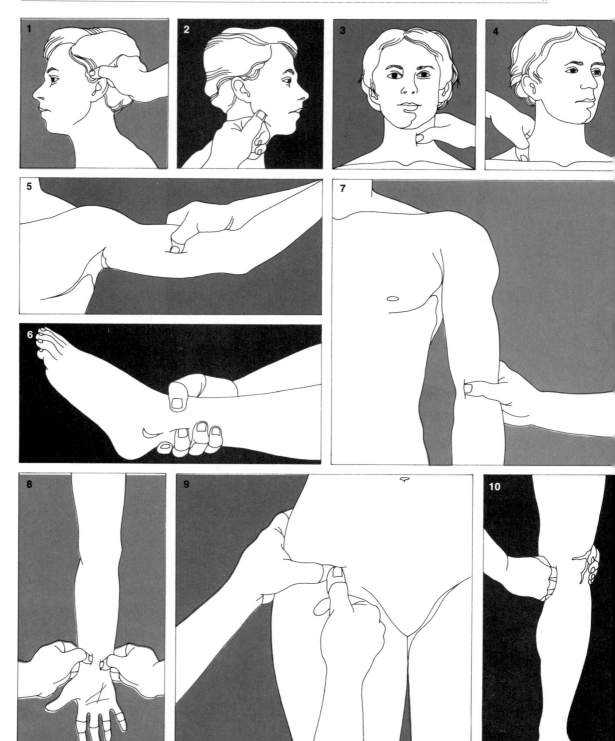

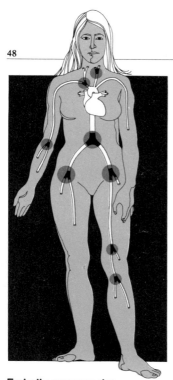

Embolic emergencies
The drawing above illustrates the common sites of embolic arterial occlusion.

if the color has changed from pink to white, suspect serious obstruction or lack of circulation. In dark-skinned patients, examine the sclera, conjunctiva, palms, or soles of the feet. Look, too, for cyanotic lips and nail beds. With severe blood loss, dark skin may have a "grayish" appearance. In less severe cases you'll find extremities cool and mottled.

• Is the patient edematous? Edema can indicate acute venous insufficiency. A cold extremity and no edema can indicate arterial insufficiency.

In cases of head injury, follow a neurologic checklist (see Chapter 12). Look for:
• confusion or restlessness
• decreased sensorium and unequal pupil size
• increased intracranial pressure with increased blood pressure and decreased pulse rate
• irregular respirations, transient paralysis, or aphasia
• bleeding from the nose, mouth or ears.

In all cases obtain the patient's history and note any serious secondary disorders such as epilepsy or diabetes that will affect the patient's care. Until you establish that a patient's injury is only external, treat it as an emergency; assess and care for him as you would a patient with an internal injury.

Treating traumatic injuries
Traumatic internal abdominal injuries can involve many organs and usually require immediate surgical intervention. How you manage the patient prior to surgery can make all the difference in his prognosis.

Two youths stabbed Ted Kronos, a letter carrier, on his way home from work. He arrived in our emergency department with the knife still protruding from his abdomen. Blood covered his clothing, and his skin was cold and clammy. To prevent further hemorrhage, we cut away his clothing, leaving the knife in place. When we took Mr. Kronos' vital signs as a baseline, we found that his blood pressure was 104/60, his radial pulses were 122, and his respirations were 28. When we checked 15 minutes later, his blood pressure had dropped to 90/50, his pulses were 130, and his respiration had increased to 30. Bilateral pulses were still present, though weak.

We also assessed him for additional wounds. Since Mr. Kronos could move both legs and had lost no feeling in them, we ruled out spinal cord injury. Mr. Kronos remained alert,

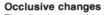

Occlusive changes

The drawings on this page show the changes in temperature and color that occlusive disease can cause. Figure 1 illustrates an occlusion of the axillary artery. Note how sharp the demarcation line is in the distal arm. Occlusions cause a significant drop in temperature and a range of color changes from mottled to blue. A saddle embolus of the aorta will produce these changes in both legs from the mid-thigh to the toes.

Figure 2 shows how an occlusion of the popliteal artery can cause changes distal to the mid-calf. An occluded femoral artery (Figure 3) will affect the distal third of the thigh.

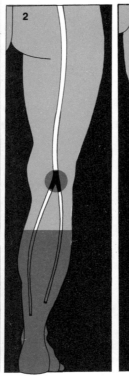

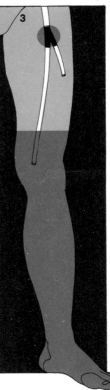

but complained of abdominal pain.

Using a large intracath, we started a rapid I.V. infusion of lactated Ringer's solution, 1000 ml, in Mr. Kronos' arm until whole blood was available. As we prepared Mr. Kronos for transfer to surgery, we inserted an additional I.V. line for CVP monitoring in his subclavian vein, using 1000 ml of lactated Ringer's solution. We drew blood for complete blood count (CBC), electrolytes, type and crossmatch. The doctor inserted a Foley catheter to assess urinary bladder injury and when we found blood in Mr. Kronos' urine, we knew he'd suffered damage to his ureters or bladder. This only increased our sense of urgency. We inserted a nasogastric tube to detect any injury and to decompress the stomach. Mr. Kronos' gastric contents showed no blood. Since the O.R. was now ready, we transferred Mr. Kronos immediately.

Many duties, little time

In emergency cases like Mr. Kronos', you must perform many duties at once to save time. Of course, first you must stop any external bleeding. Then, as you take vital signs, you can also assess respiratory status and look for additional wounds. Since we didn't know if a major abdominal vessel was involved, we didn't start I.V. fluid in either lower extremity. To do so would have risked extravasating fluid into Mr. Kronos' abdominal cavity or retroperitoneal space. Correspondingly, if Mr. Kronos' neck area had been involved, we wouldn't have started an I.V. in the upper extremities.

Notice that we made no attempt to restore Mr. Kronos' blood volume or vital signs to normal. Although we did replace some of the fluid volume lost, we knew that infusing blood and administering vasoconstrictors to maintain systolic blood pressure waste valuable time. Under these conditions, Mr. Kronos would have lost the blood as quickly as it was infused, and raising his blood pressure would only have contributed to this.

With patients in better condition than Mr. Kronos, you may have time to get a preop chest X-ray and an intravenous pyelogram (IVP) to assess any genitourinary injury. The patient may also need tetanus, as well as antibiotic prophylaxis. However, if the injury has lacerated a major abdominal vessel, you should rush the patient to surgery immediately to avoid exsanguination.

The saddle embolus

Not all vascular emergencies involve hemorrhage. Degenerative disease, such as atherosclerosis, may cause acute arterial occlusion from thrombosis or embolism, ruptured abdominal aneurysm, or acute dissecting aneurysm—any of which endanger the patient's life.

Consider 55-year-old Simon Keefe, a patient with a history of myocardial infarction and mitral stenosis. He came to the E.D. complaining of sudden severe pain in both legs, then loss of feeling. When we examined him, we found his legs cool and mottled, and his toenail beds cyanotic. No palpable pulses were present in his groin or ankles. We asked him about his pain and how rapidly his symptoms had developed. Then we called the doctor immediately since we suspected an embolus, probably at the bifurcation of the aorta (a saddle embolus). Emergency arteriography confirmed our suspicions, and Mr. Keefe was rushed to surgery.

Obstruction in the extremities, like Mr. Keefe's, can suggest acute venous thrombosis, which generally occurs in deep veins, but we ruled this out because of his history and because of the sudden onset of his symptoms. This suddenness suggests an acute arterial embolism rather than chronic arterial insufficiency. In chronic arterial insufficiency, Mr. Keefe would have suffered a slowly progressing coolness and discoloration below the obstruction. (See page 48 for common sites of arterial obstructions.) He might first have noticed pain while walking (intermittent claudication), because of increased tissue demand for blood. Then, as circulatory obstruction increased, he'd have suffered pain, even at rest.

Assessing aneurysms

Arteriosclerosis or atherosclerosis can cause an artery to dilate, weakening the arterial wall. The condition is called an aneurysm. Aneurysms develop mostly in the abdominal aorta but can also form in a cerebral, thoracic, femoral, popliteal, or any large artery. An abdominal aneurysm feels like a pulsating swelling in the abdomen. On an X-ray it may look like a shadow outlined by calcium. The patient's femoral pulses remain palpable, which distinguishes an abdominal aneurysm from an embolus in the abdominal aorta. The patient may have back pain and abdominal discomfort, or he may be asymptomatic.

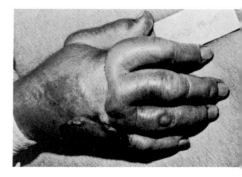

Winter's sting

In areas where winter weather is severe, prolonged exposure to cold can damage a patient's face, nose, ears, hands, and feet. How serious the injury is depends on wind velocity, temperature, humidity, and the kind and duration of exposure.

Frostbite occurs when the tissue actually freezes. The patient may not even realize he's been injured until he returns to a warm place and suffers severe burning pain. The affected part may be numb and may appear pale white and glossy or even blistered, as in burn injuries. Edema may hamper the palpation of peripheral pulses.

Rewarm the part in tepid (99° to 103° F.) water. When the part begins to thaw, the patient will feel a tingling sensation. Reexamine the extremities for pulses and then wrap the part in a bulky sterile dressing. But don't rub the part, because you can aggravate the damage. If the patient's feet are involved, don't let him walk. Make sure you place cotton or gauze sponges between his toes to prevent maceration.

Doctors commonly prescribe lidocaine or papaverine to reduce the vasospasms that cold injuries cause. They also order antibiotics and tetanus prophylaxis.

A tight squeeze
Antishock trousers counteract bleeding and shock and may be applied to treat an abdominal aneurysm rupture. How do they work? When applied to the patient's legs and abdomen and inflated, the special polyvinyl pants' accumulated pressure compresses the patient's peripheral circulation under the trousers. As the pressure exceeds the patient's systolic blood pressure, pooled venous blood in the patient's legs and abdomen returns to his central circulation. This, in turn, slows or reverses the hemorrhage or shock.

Suppose the aneurysm ruptures? Suspect this if the patient has sudden, severe back and abdominal pain and symptoms of shock. *Get help immediately, or the patient will bleed to death.* Alert the O.R., then with the help of other staff members, complete the following priorities *stat:* Check vital signs; start lactated Ringer's solution I.V. (using a large-bore catheter); draw blood for type and crossmatch and measurements of blood gases; have a Foley catheter inserted to measure urine output, and then rush the patient to surgery.

An acute dissecting aneurysm generally occurs in the ascending thoracic aorta. A tear in the intima will cause blood to penetrate between the linings of the artery. The blood collects in a sac that blocks the artery, stopping circulation below the dissection.

When a patient has this type of aneurysm he usually complains of agonizing pain in his upper back and may show symptoms of shock. These symptoms are confusingly similar to those of a myocardial infarction. Try to distinguish them quickly, however, because as the dissection progresses, the patient will deteriorate rapidly as the loosened intima blocks the aorta. Watch for paralysis or hemiplegia, the absence of peripheral pulses, and a difference in blood pressure on the affected side. The development of an aortic diastolic murmur will help diagnose the condition accurately. Remember, deep breathing or changing position will not increase the patient's pain. As the dissection progresses, though, the pain may shift from the original site to a lower portion of the chest. An acute dissecting aneurysm is managed similarly to a ruptured abdominal aneurysm. Your quick assessment and speedy treatment can help save the patient's life.

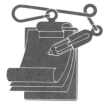

Remember these important points when caring for a patient with a vascular emergency:
1. Control bleeding by using the appropriate pressure point.
2. Determine hemorrhage severity by the type, number, and location of vessels involved.
3. Recognize arterial hemorrhage by the way blood spurts out with each pulsation.
4. Antishock trousers increase the patient's circulatory volume faster than I.V. replacement fluids.

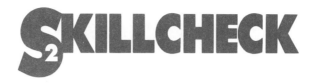

SKILLCHECK

1. You've just finished working an 8-hour shift in the surgical unit of a hospital and are on your way home. Suddenly, you remember that you're out of yogurt and stop at a supermarket just 6 blocks from your apartment. As you push your shopping cart down the aisle where the dairy products are located, you see an elderly woman gasp, clutch at her chest, and fall to the floor. What do you do next?

2. Virgil Rippy is a 48-year-old engraver who has recovered well after undergoing surgery for cancer of the larynx. As a rehabilitated laryngectomee, and member of the Lost Chord Club (American Laryngectomy Association), Mr. Rippy frequently comes to the hospital to counsel patients undergoing this type of surgery. One day, he doesn't look well to you. But before you can ask him what is wrong, he loses consciousness and collapses at your feet. What do you do?

3. One cold night, Frank Potenick is rushed to the emergency department with severe chest pains. According to his wife — who accompanied him to the hospital — Mr. Potenick started having episodes of pain earlier in the evening, after shoveling their snow-covered driveway. He looks extremely pale, is having difficulty breathing, and is diaphoretic. He gasps that he's afraid and doesn't want his wife to leave his side. What do you do next?

4. You're a nurse in a CCU. The lab has just called to report the initial cardiac enzyme levels for George Baylor — a patient who has just been admitted with a possible myocardial infarction. All of his signs and symptoms so far suggest that he's suffered an MI, but the lab tells you that his cardiac enzyme levels are normal. Can the lab report be wrong?

5. Minutes after you arrive for a barbecue supper at your neighbor's house, her 2-year-old son Jimmy is discovered floating face-down in the backyard swimming pool. By the time you reach the pool, the child has been pulled out of the water and another guest has begun giving artificial respiration. You tell the child's mother to call an ambulance, then you offer your assistance to the rescuer — explaining first that you're a nurse. As you stoop to help, you notice that Jimmy's stomach is becoming markedly distended. What do you do?

6. Three victims of a gas-main explosion are brought into the emergency department on the day you're doing triage. They had been shopping in a grocery store when the explosion occurred and a plate glass window shattered, injuring everyone nearby. A quick check tells you that each of the victims has multiple lacerations over his entire body. As triage nurse, how can you determine which patient needs priority treatment?

7. For the past six weeks, you've been working in the emergency department of a small rural hospital. You've just finished giving immediate aid to a woman with a Japanese beetle lodged in her ear, when 35-year-old LeRoy Thompson is brought in with severe injuries suffered in a farm accident. His father, who has accompanied him, tells you that Mr. Thompson's left hand and forearm got caught in a piece of farm equipment and were badly mangled. The three towels that are wrapped around Mr. Thompson's arm are saturated with blood. What do you do first?

8. Eighteen-year-old Jake Justus went backpacking with two friends one weekend and accidentally slashed his right forearm with his hunting knife. To stop the severe hemorrhaging that resulted from the deep laceration, one of the boys applied a tourniquet to Jake's arm, just above his elbow. By the time they reach the emergency department where you are a nurse, Jake's arm has stopped bleeding. What do you do?

(Answers on page 181)

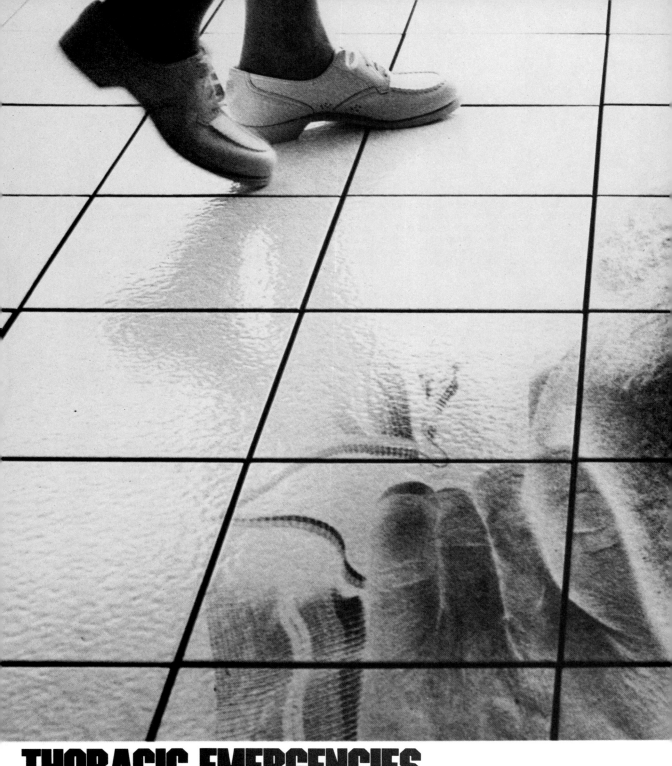

THORACIC EMERGENCIES

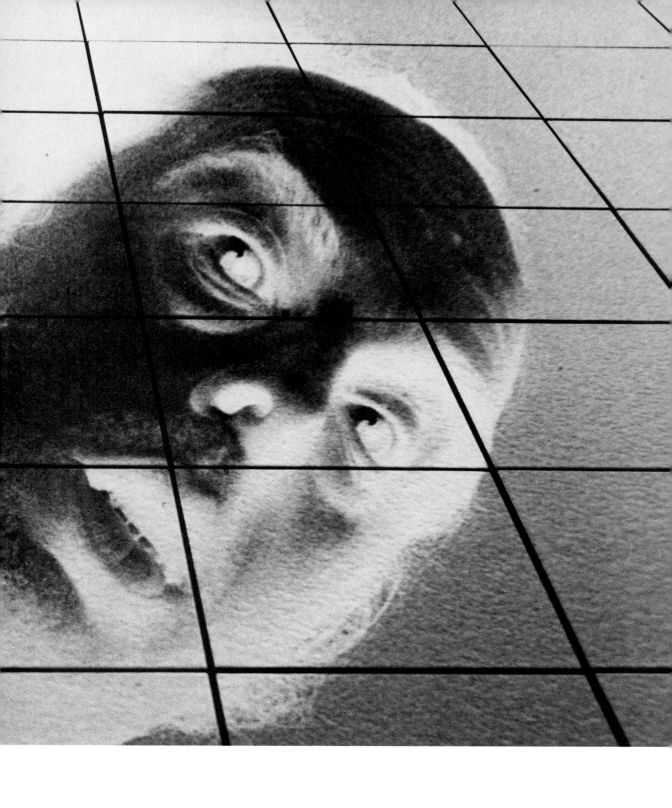

When would you expect the doctor to order
rotating tourniquets for a patient?

If you deliver a high percentage of oxygen to a
patient with chronic asthma, what may occur?

When a patient sustains a penetrating chest
wound, what are your emergency care
priorities?

What signs and symptoms indicate
cardiac tamponade?

When is surgery indicated in a patient
with lung trauma?

6

Respiratory Crisis
How to combat severe breathing difficulties

MARGARET F. FUHS, RN, MSN

YOU'RE DOING TRIAGE in the emergency department of a big city hospital when ambulance attendants wheel in the unconscious victim of a construction accident. His injuries seem severe, but suddenly they're not your primary concern. Why? Because the patient has vomited, obstructing his airway.

Airway obstruction, of course, is a respiratory emergency, which means it takes precedence over all others. With respiratory arrest, irreversible brain damage and death occur in just a few minutes — unless you immediately restore the patient's breathing.

But airway obstruction — which I'll review for you on the following two pages — isn't the only respiratory emergency a patient may have. You'll probably see other problems that require priority care. For example, a patient may come to the hospital with acute pulmonary edema, or some form of acute exacerbation of chronic obstructive pulmonary disease (COPD). Or he may have serious respiratory complications from a near-drowning accident.

What do you know about these critical conditions? Could you tell if a patient had status asthmaticus? What about pulmonary emphysema or chronic bronchitis? What kind of

Opening the obstructed airway

Sudden airway obstruction can be caused by a foreign body in the throat or bronchus; laryngeal or vocal cord edema; aspiration of blood, mucus, or vomitus; the tongue's falling against the pharynx; traumatic injury; or bronchoconstriction or bronchospasm.

With complete obstruction, anoxia will cause death in approximately 3 to 5 minutes—unless breathing is restored.

As you know from Chapter 3, the head-tilt–neck-lift or head-tilt–chin-lift methods may be enough to open the airway in a supine patient. But suppose his airway is obstructed by vomitus, blood, mucus, or a foreign body? If this happens, try to remove the obstruction quickly by using the following maneuvers:

If the patient's mouth is closed, force it open immediately using the crossed-finger technique shown in Figure 1. To do this properly, place your thumb on the patient's lower teeth and your index finger on his upper teeth at the corner of his mouth. Force downward with your thumb and upward with your index finger. Hold the mouth open.

Nursing tip: If the patient has poor fitting dentures, remove these at once so they don't slip out of place and further obstruct his airway (see Figure 2).

Now turn the patient's head to one side, or logroll him in the proper way, if you suspect he has a spinal injury. Insert your index and middle fingers deep into his throat and try to remove the obstruction, if it's visible, by sweeping out his oral cavity, as shown in Figure 3.

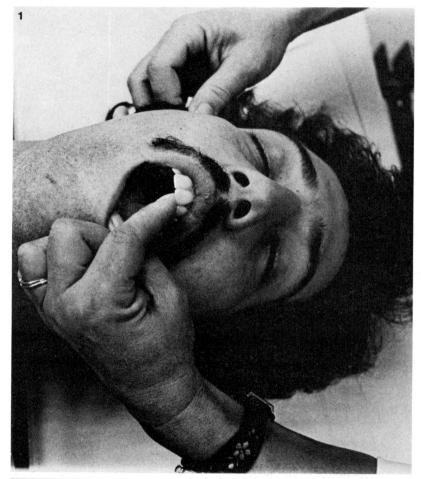

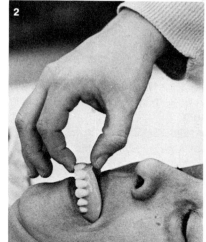

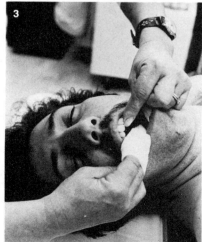

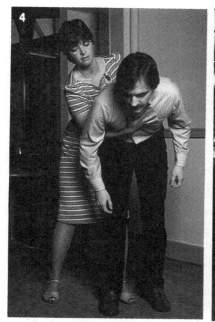

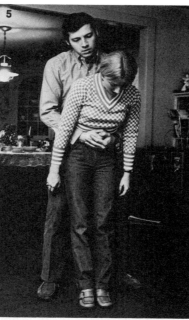

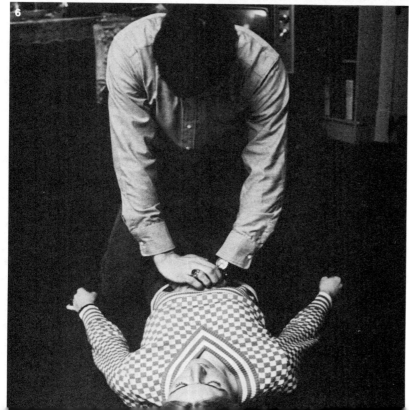

Or use suctioning equipment.

If you are unable to dislodge the obstruction, roll the patient toward you. Then, using the heel of your hand, deliver 4 sharp blows between his shoulder blades (see Figure 4).

The abdominal thrust
If the sharp back blows fail to dislodge the object, use the abdominal thrust maneuver. You can use this on a standing patient, as well as one who remains supine.

With a standing patient, wrap your arms around her waist, as shown in Figure 5. Place your fist with the thumb side against the patient's epigastrium, grasp your fist with your other hand, and press upward with a quick thrust. Repeat 4 times.

With a supine patient, kneel astride her hips as shown in Figure 6, and place your hands, one on top of the other, over her epigastrium. With the heel of your bottom hand, press upward with a quick thrust. Repeat 4 times.

Now look into the victim's mouth and attempt a finger sweep only if the obstructing object is visible

If the abdominal thrust is ineffective, attempt to ventilate the patient and then give him 4 more back blows, followed by 4 abdominal thrusts.

Once you've cleared the patient's airway, restore breathing with artificial respiration. If you can't get an open airway using any of the above techniques, the patient may require endotracheal intubation or a cricothyreotomy. Most doctors would rather not perform a tracheostomy under emergency conditions.

Trach tips
Here's how to care for the patient with a new tracheostomy:
1. Tie the strings that hold the outer tube in place around the patient's neck. They should be secure, yet loose enough to allow for possible swelling.
2. Watch the stomal site for bleeding or irritation. Place an unfrayed sterile dressing around the collar of the tracheostomy tube.
3. Position the patient for comfort and easy breathing.
4. Have an obturator and another tracheostomy tube (same size) at the bedside and the proper suctioning equipment nearby.
5. Reassure the patient. Make sure he knows he won't be able to speak normally. Have the paper, pencil, call bell, and any other necessary communication materials within easy reach at the bedside. Put a note by the intercom informing everyone that the patient can't speak. Then tell him you've done this so he won't be anxious.

emergency care should each of these patients have? Seconds count, you know. The wrong move on your part may cost the patient his life.

I'll review all of these emergencies for you in this chapter, starting with airway obstruction. Then I'll give you the care priorities you should follow for each, so you can work with speed and effectiveness.

Getting down to basics

As you know, the respiratory system uses the processes of ventilation, perfusion, and diffusion for one important function—to deliver oxygen to, and remove carbon dioxide from, body cells. If the patient develops a respiratory disorder, any or all of these processes may be affected.

Depending on the disorder, the patient may hyperventilate or hypoventilate—either of which disrupts the normal oxygen and/or carbon dioxide levels in his blood. When a patient hyperventilates, too much air is moved in and out of his alveoli in too short a time. This causes abnormal loss of carbon dioxide and results in alkalosis. On the other hand, when a patient hypoventilates, too little air is moved in and out of his alveoli in a given time. This keeps normal gas exchange from taking place; in other words, not enough oxygen gets into the blood and not enough carbon dioxide gets removed. Acid levels in the blood rise, resulting in acidosis.

To properly assess respiratory function, the doctor must study the patient's arterial blood gas levels at regular intervals. Examine the normal levels on page 62. Respiratory failure occurs when the blood's carbon dioxide level is 50 mm Hg or more, and/or the oxygen level is 50 mm Hg or less.

Pulmonary edema

Now let's talk about some of the conditions that seriously affect respiratory function: for example, pulmonary edema.

Pulmonary edema occurs when fluid passes from the pulmonary capillaries into the alveoli. The most common cause for this fluid shift is left ventricular impairment, which increases left pulmonary artery pressure—as well as pressure in the pulmonary veins and capillaries. As a general rule, anytime pulmonary artery pressure rises above 35 mm Hg, fluid passes into the alveoli rapidly.

As I said, left ventricular heart failure is the most common cause of pulmonary edema. But other conditions of noncardiac origin may also trigger it. For example, a patient may develop pulmonary edema from pulmonary emboli, renal failure, toxic gas inhalation, or ingestion and aspiration of toxic substances.

Looking at Mr. Preston's case
How can you tell when a patient develops pulmonary edema? And what can you do about it? To illustrate, consider the case of 63-year-old Harold Preston, who's rushed to the E.D. with severe dyspnea. As you place him in a high-Fowler's position, you note and record the following signs and symptoms on your assessment sheet:
• labored, noisy breathing with wheezing on inspiration and expiration
• use of accessory muscles to breathe
• neck vein distention
• diaphoresis and anxiety
• cyanotic lips and nail beds
• productive cough with pink-tinged, frothy sputum.
Continuing with your assessment, you auscultate Mr. Preston's chest and discover diffuse bilateral rales. His vital signs are: blood pressure 190/114, pulse 134, and respiratory rate 36.

When you ask Mr. Preston how long he's been having trouble breathing, he tells you that his symptoms started several weeks ago. He's had trouble sleeping, because he starts coughing in his sleep and wakes up unable to catch his breath. "Sometimes I have to sit up all night in a chair," he gasps, "just...so...I...can...breathe...comfortably."

A further look at Mr. Preston's medical history reveals that he suffered a severe myocardial infarction 5 years earlier and has had periodic anginal attacks ever since. He's been taking nitroglycerin sublingually for the angina and usually receives prompt relief.

The doctor's evaluation indicates Mr. Preston's pulmonary edema comes from left ventricular failure. So you'll treat him with digitalis and diuretics to improve left ventricular function, and reduce fluid overload. The doctor may also order rotating tourniquets to retard venous return to right side of heart.

After your initial assessment and the doctor's evaluation have been completed, he'll most likely order this plan of care:

Normal adult ranges for arterial blood gases
pH   7.35 to 7.45
PCO_2 35 to 45 mm Hg
HCO   22 to 26 mEq/liter
PO_2 75 to 100 mm Hg
O_2 94% to 100%

• Administer oxygen by face mask at a high liter flow to reverse hypoxia and relieve dyspnea. If ventilation remains hindered by fluid in lungs, switch to intermittent positive-pressure breathing (IPPB) to provide counter-pressure against existing pressure in pulmonary capillaries. *Caution:* Watch the patient closely. IPPB can decrease venous return to his right atrium, causing his blood pressure to drop rapidly.

• If the patient isn't allergic to morphine, give 10 mg of this drug by slow I.V. push. Morphine will decrease ineffective respiratory effort and alleviate some of the patient's extreme anxiety. *Caution:* Never give morphine to a patient with co-existing COPD or cardiogenic shock. As you know, morphine depresses respirations and may cause the shock patient's blood pressure to drop even further.

Whenever you give morphine, watch the patient's respirations closely and keep naloxone HCl (Narcan) 400 mcg—a morphine antagonist—nearby.

• Administer aminophylline (500 mg I.V. diluted in 50 ml of 5% dextrose in water) over a period of 15 minutes to open alveoli and improve ventilation. *Nursing tip:* When you give the drug over this period of time, you reduce the risk of sudden drop in blood pressure, syncope, and possible death from rapid systemic vasodilation.

• Administer digoxin 0.5 mg I.V. to begin digitalization of the patient. (The dosage would be different, of course, if the patient had been taking digoxin at home.)

• Administer furosemide (Lasix) 40 mg by slow I.V. push to promote diuresis and alleviate the symptoms caused by fluid overload. Additional furosemide may be needed to relieve symptoms. Begin keeping an intake/output record to help manage fluid balance.

• Take a 3- to 5-lead EKG to check for recent damage to the heart.

• Try to relieve the patient's anxiety by staying with him, reassuring him, and explaining every procedure.

Always keep an emergency endotracheal intubation tray handy when you're caring for a patient with pulmonary edema. Remember, if the relatively conservative measure I've outlined above fails, you may have to treat the patient with rotating tourniquets and a respirator. (For full details on how rotating tourniquets are applied to decrease blood flow to right heart and lungs, see pages 64 to 65.)

COPD: Asthma, emphysema, and chronic bronchitis
We use the term chronic obstructive pulmonary disease (COPD) to group together three disorders: asthma, emphysema, and chronic bronchitis. All three disorders have one condition in common: obstruction of the small airways, generally the bronchioles. Clinically, these disorders are grouped because they can be difficult to separate. A patient may suffer symptoms and complications from two or even all three. *A reminder:* COPD is sometimes referred to by these terms: chronic airway obstruction (CAO) and chronic obstructive lung disease (COLD).

Asthma: When allergy narrows the airways
If you work in the emergency department, you've probably cared for a patient like Louise Brady. For years, Mrs. Brady has suffered from allergic asthma—a condition characterized by obstruction of the bronchioles. What causes this obstruction? A narrowing of the bronchioles from spasms; scant, thick mucous secretion; and edema.

Shortly after lunch one day, frail Mrs. Brady is rushed to the E.D. by her terrified daughter. You see at once that Mrs. Brady looks even more terrified. She's so short of breath that she's clutching at her neck to loosen her clothing and using all her accessory muscles to breathe.

"My mother has had attacks like this before," Mrs. Brady's daughter tells you. But now the attacks occur with greater frequency. When Mrs. Brady first developed asthma, she remained symptom-free between attacks, but now she has chronic dyspnea. Earlier in the week, Mrs. Brady was troubled by her usual shortness of breath, inspiratory and expiratory wheezing, and a non-productive, irritating cough. Suddenly, her condition became much worse, so when her regular medication failed to relieve her bronchospasms, her daughter rushed her to the hospital.

What can you do for a patient like Mrs. Brady? The doctor will probably order the following:
• Place her in semi-Fowler's position, reassure her that you will help her, and urge her to relax as much as possible.
• Administer oxygen by nasal cannula at 2 liters/minute until you can obtain the results of arterial blood-gas measurements. Adjust oxygen concentration, as needed.

Caution: Never administer a high percentage of oxygen

Rotating tourniquets

You're caring for a 35-year-old man with acute pulmonary edema. Prescribed drug therapy isn't bringing results, and the patient's condition worsens. The doctor turns to you and says, "Get him on the automatic rotating tourniquets, *stat*."

Would you be ready for that order? How long is it since you used an automatic rotating tourniquet machine?

Phlebotomy, potent diuretics, and digoxin have diminished the use of automatic rotating tourniquets. But when drugs and bleeding fail, or when you're waiting for them to take effect, you may have to get out the automatic rotating tourniquets. And when the need arises, the situation is apt to be critical. As you know, acute pulmonary edema occurs most commonly in patients with heart disease, hypertension, arteriosclerosis, and fluid overload. It can be caused by left ventricular failure, high altitude, inhaled materials, narcotic overdose, or renal failure. It usually comes on abruptly.

Doctors ordinarily order the use of rotating tourniquets for patients with congestive heart failure. Rotating tourniquets decrease the circulating blood volume by entrapping fluid in the extremities. Venous return and right ventricular output decrease, which help decongest the lungs.

When you explain the procedure and its purpose to the patient (Figure 1), tell him that the skin of the extremities may become discolored so he won't be anxious. Then take his blood pressure as a base line.

When applying the tourniquets, place them over a small towel as high as possible on three extremities. Leave one extremity free each time. To make sure that you haven't occluded the arterial vessels, check to see that you can place two fingers between the tourniquet cuff and the padding

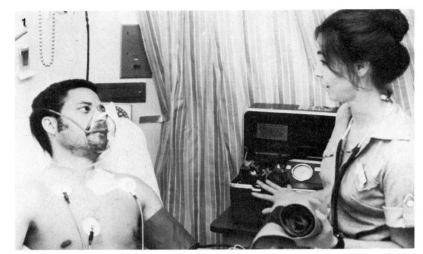

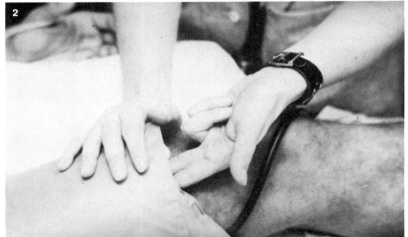

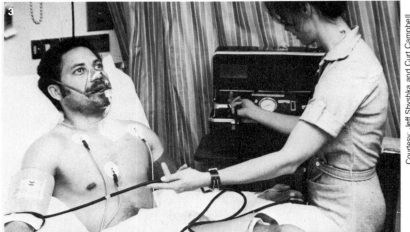

Courtesy: Jeff Shyshka and Curt Campbell

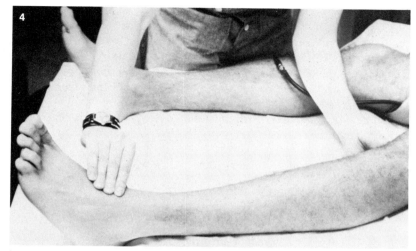

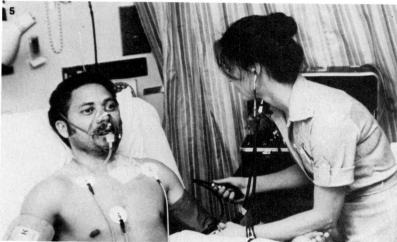

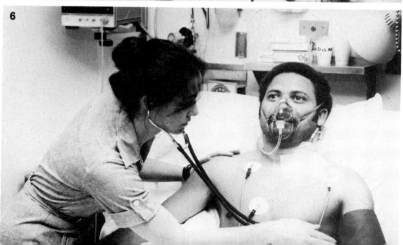

(Figure 2). As an additional check, feel for the arterial pulse in the tied extremity.

Release one tourniquet every 15 minutes and apply it to the previously free extremity, following a clockwise rotation. You can safely occlude the venous outflow in any single extremity for 45 minutes, except on elderly patients or those with poor circulation. For these patients, rotate the tourniquets every 5 minutes to prevent complications.

Regularly check the cuffs to make sure they're not too tight (Figure 3) and the extremities for adequate pulses (Figure 4). The use of tourniquets precipitates hypotension in some patients.

When releasing the tourniquets, remove them one at a time at 15-minute intervals to avoid a recurrence of pulmonary edema. Check the patient's blood pressure after removing a cuff (Figure 5) and then check his lungs and heart sounds for any irregularities (Figure 6).

Prolonged or excessive tourniquet pressures are likely to cause damage to the blood vessels; thrombophlebitis; laceration, softening, or necrosis of the tissues; metabolic acidosis, a shift in the acid/base status of the body; pulmonary emboli; or myocardial infarction.

If your patient has a tendency toward hemorrhage, tourniquets can cause bleeding. If he has peripheral blood clots, tourniquets can increase their size and stop blood flow. And if such a clot is dislodged, it could threaten the heart, lungs, kidneys, or brain. Other contraindications are a preexistent infection or ischemia, impairment of the right atrium, shock or impending shock, or peripheral vascular disease.

The doctor (and you, too) must balance the benefits against the potential risks of using tourniquets.

(above 40%) to a patient with chronic asthma or another form of COPD. If you do, she may stop breathing. The reason for this is simple: A normal person breathes because his respiratory system is stimulated by an increased carbon dioxide level. Because the patient with chronic asthma may consistently retain a high level of carbon dioxide, her respiratory center can get narcotized and hypoxia can become her only stimulus for breathing. As you can see, administering a high percentage of oxygen could then depress her hypoxic drive and cause her to stop breathing.

• Be sure to start an I.V. of 5% dextrose in water to hydrate the patient.

• Administer the bronchodilator, aminophylline (500 mg I.V. in 100 ml of 5% dextrose in water) over a period of 20 minutes, and the anti-inflammatory drug, hydrocortisone (Solu-Cortef) 100 mg I.V. to reduce bronchospasm, as ordered. In addition, the doctor may also order epinephrine (Adrenalin) 1:1,000 solution, 0.5 ml subcutaneously every 20 minutes for three doses to help relax the patient's bronchial muscles.

• Have an arterial blood sample drawn to measure blood-gas levels. If your patient is receiving oxygen, be sure to note it on the lab slip. (Mrs. Brady's blood-gas levels indicated an elevated PO_2 and PCO_2.) The PO_2 reflects hypoxia. The elevated PCO_2 reflects hypoventilation. A patient with chronic asthma—as well as one with pure emphysema—normally maintains PCO_2 at normal or subnormal levels for years by hyperventilating during acute episodes. However, when her condition becomes so severe that she tires, she hypoventilates and acidosis occurs. An asthmatic who's still hyperventilating may come in with hypocarbia (decreased carbon dioxide in the blood), which will result in alkalosis.

• Always obtain arterial blood-gas measurements as soon as possible, so you can treat the existing condition effectively. Remember, epinephrine—which is usually used for acute asthma—is inactivated by acidosis. You must reverse acidosis by ventilation and sodium bicarbonate I.V. before administering epinephrine.

Status asthmaticus
Though an acute asthmatic attack frightens the patient and requires immediate care, it's usually reversible with proper treatment and sometimes reverses spontaneously. However,

when the usual therapy becomes ineffective, the condition progresses to status asthmaticus.

With status asthmaticus, the patient develops increased dyspnea and will need aggressive emergency treatment to keep her bronchioles from becoming completely obstructed. She'll probably appear even more terrified than the usual asthmatic patient because of her difficulty breathing. She may not even wheeze, she'll be taking in so little air. And her neck veins may show distention because of increased pulmonary artery pressure.

Unless the patient has a known history of asthma, you may mistake status asthmaticus for another chronic obstructive lung disease or even pulmonary edema. However, when status asthmaticus is the diagnosis, the doctor will probably order the treatment usually used to reverse an acute asthma attack. If this fails, he may order isoproterenol (Isuprel) 1:200 diluted in warm saline solution, administered with a positive-pressure breathing machine. He may also order a broad-spectrum antibiotic, because status asthmaticus may be triggered by severe lung infection. Few doctors use bronchoscopy with bronchial lavage because the procedure can cause further bronchospasms. *Caution:* Be prepared to put the patient on a respirator if she goes into complete respiratory failure.

Remember these important tips when you give emergency care for a patient with status asthmaticus:

• Don't confuse the tachycardia usually present with this condition with a dangerous arrhythmia. Status asthmaticus tachycardia generally results from anxiety and the administration of sympathomimetic drugs, and requires no treatment.

• Don't attempt to relieve the patient's anxiety with narcotics or sedatives. These drugs will further depress respirations.

• Don't hyperventilate the patient to the point of alkalosis. To prevent this, have blood-gas levels measured at regular intervals.

Emphysema and chronic bronchitis
As I mentioned earlier, the patient with COPD may also have emphysema or chronic bronchitis. These conditions, although worrisome to the patient, only become emergencies when there's acute exacerbation.

The emphasematous patient is usually thin and looks pink, but his heart shows little or no enlargement and his cough

Fitting a face mask

Anyone who has tried, knows that fitting an Ambu mask properly can be tricky. To begin, use both hands to spread the edges of the mask laterally. Then, as the mask returns to its original shape, it will gather up the flesh, making a tighter seal (Figures 1 and 2).

Don't worry about air escaping around the patient's face as long as you can see an adequate rise and fall of the chest. If the bag collapses completely with each squeeze, it will provide the patient with an adequate tidal volume even though a lot of air is wasted.

To hold the mask in place, use your non-dominant hand (your left if you are right-handed). Place your fingers under the patient's chin to keep his head in position (Figure 3). If you use this method, your dominant hand will be free to squeeze the bag and to operate suction equipment, if necessary, between breaths (Figure 4). Do not use face masks with straps to keep them on tight. These endanger the patient since he will almost certainly aspirate if he vomits while the mask is strapped in place.

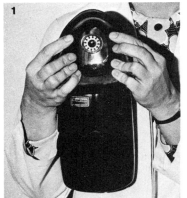

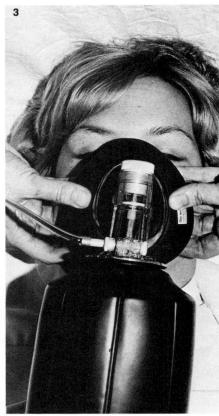

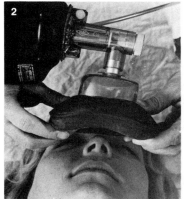

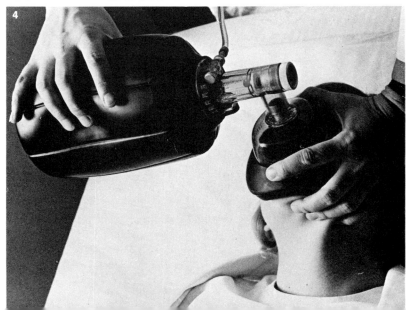

produces little sputum. He may be hypoxic, but — like the asthmatic patient — doesn't retain carbon dioxide, so he may not be acidotic. His difficulties arise from permanent over-inflation of the bronchioles and lung tissue destruction. This patient has more air in his lungs than he needs, resulting in the familiar "barrel chest."

In chronic bronchitis, the bronchial mucosa gets inflamed and edematous, narrowing the air passages. When this happens, the mucus glands throughout the trachea and bronchi overproduce mucus. Pure bronchitis causes hypoxia and carbon dioxide retention. The patient, who is usually heavy-set, looks reddish-blue, has ankle edema, and distended neck veins. His reddish-blue appearance indicates polycythemia, which is the body's attempt to compensate for the decreased oxygen in the red blood cells.

When you see a patient with emphysema or chronic bronchitis in the E.D., he's usually struggling to breathe. His temperature may be elevated; he'll probably be diaphoretic and extremely anxious. Following the doctor's orders, work quickly to relieve the patient's anxiety and dyspnea. Place him in a comfortable position and start treating him with low percentage, low-flow oxygen, I.V. fluids, bronchodilators, an aerosol medication like isoproterenol (using a positive-pressure breathing machine). Add antibiotics and expectorants to the drug regimen, if the doctor orders them for suspected pulmonary infection. And watch for changes that may indicate respiratory failure.

The near-drowning victim
The last condition that I want to talk about in this chapter is the victim of a near-drowning accident. He may or may not be unconscious when admitted to the E.D., and he'll probably show the signs and symptoms of asphyxia and pulmonary edema: for example, cyanosis, frothy sputum, tachypnea, tachycardia, and rales.

To give quick and effective emergency care to this patient, the doctor will probably order this care:

• Establish and maintain an open airway and administer oxygen at a low percentage until you can obtain blood-gas measurements.

• Have a nasogastric tube inserted to remove swallowed air and fluid from the patient's stomach.

- Have an arterial blood sample drawn to measure blood-gas levels, and get a venous blood sample to measure electrolytes.
- Metabolic and respiratory acidosis are usually present because of carbon dioxide retention and oxygen depletion. Be ready to give sodium bicarbonate I.V.
- Start an I.V. with the appropriate solution. Which solution you use depends on the patient's blood volume and electrolyte levels. When a patient has nearly drowned in fresh water, the introduction of a hypotonic solution to his system causes increased blood volume (as it diffuses into the capillaries), resulting in electrolyte dilution. Conversely, when a patient has nearly drowned in salt water, the introduction of a hypertonic solution to his system decreases blood volume, resulting in electrolyte concentration.
- Watch the patient closely for signs of increased respiratory distress. A near-drowning victim should be hospitalized for at least 48 hours, so that prompt action can be taken if he develops pulmonary edema.

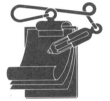

Remember these important points when caring for a patient in respiratory crisis:

1. Attempt to clear an airway obstruction by using back blows, abdominal or chest thrusts, finger sweeps (in this order).

2. Administer a low percentage of oxygen (under 40%), as needed, to a patient with chronic asthma or other form of COPD.

3. Take nursing measures to relieve anxiety in a patient with status asthmaticus. Never give narcotics or sedatives.

4. Carefully assess a near-drowning victim for signs of pulmonary edema.

5. Before sending an arterial blood sample to the lab, note on the lab slip if the patient is receiving oxygen.

6. Position rotating tourniquets as high as possible on three extremities. Place each tourniquet over a small towel. Be aware of the potential risks of rotating tourniquets.

7

Chest Trauma
What to do in the first critical minutes

EDWARD LANCE, MD
AND HANNELORE SWEETWOOD, RN, BS

CHEST TRAUMA CALLS FOR an exception to usual nursing routine. You may have to shoot first and ask questions later. Sure, under normal circumstances, you'd include a history and a brief physical examination as part of your assessment. Not so with chest trauma victims. Every minute counts. Your ability to make a rapid assessment of the patient and the extent of his injury will form the basis for the treatment — and for whatever lifesaving decisions have to be made.

Top priority: The airway
Let's take the case of 21-year-old John LaVerne, who was repairing his roof when he fell off the ladder and landed on his picket fence. He's rushed to the emergency department, and when you see him he's bleeding heavily from a wound in his chest.

What do you do first? Try to control the bleeding? No, you ignore it — no matter how severe — until you make sure John has an open airway.

Providing an open airway and temporarily occluding any thoracic wounds are always the first order of business. This means deferring the treatment of bleeding, shock, and other

Where is the wound?

When assessing chest wounds, try to imagine what organs or vessels may have been damaged — based upon your knowledge of thoracic anatomy.

The scapula usually comes to the level of the seventh rib posteriorly. The dome of the diaphragm on the right usually reaches the level of the fifth rib anteriorly and on the left to the level of the sixth rib anteriorly. The left ventricle usually lies medial to the nipple line anteriorly with the apex in the fifth intercostal space in the midclavicular line.

The apices of the lung often extend above the clavicle bilaterally and the subclavian vessels lie closely related to the clavicle. Thus, it can be seen, that injuries at the base of the neck may cause a pneumothorax. Anterior injuries below the level of the fifth rib on the right may affect the liver and below the sixth rib on the left may affect the spleen.

less threatening emergencies until you're sure the patient is breathing adequately.

How can you assess ventilation rapidly? We recommend a simple maneuver — first formulated by Rutherford and Gott in 1968 — which will allow you to detect most immediately life-threatening disturbances of cardiopulmonary function. To accomplish the maneuver, place your ear close to John's mouth and nose. Simultaneously watch his chest movements and palpate his carotid pulse. Gauge the force and duration of the expired air blown against your ear. A strong airflow indicates a clear airway; a poor airflow, despite an apparently strong effort, probably indicates obstruction. And, of course, absence of both pulse and airflow indicates cardiopulmonary arrest. (For a complete discussion of cardiopulmonary resuscitation techniques, see Chapter 3; see Chapter 6 for information on airway obstruction.)

Looking for wounds

John's airway is open, so you turn your attention to his thoracic injury. Cut off his clothing and examine his back and his chest — looking for any penetrating wounds that may be there from the picket fence. *Use your ears as well as your eyes;* if John has a so-called sucking wound, you'll probably hear it before you see it. Sucking wounds, of course, are life-threatening. They destroy the pressure gradient between the atmosphere and the pleural space; unless quickly restored, this loss leads to pneumothorax, mediastinal shift, and then complete respiratory failure.

Act fast. Close John's wound as quickly as possible with a gauze bandage made airtight with a petroleum jelly coating. The best time to apply the bandage: at the end of maximum expiration when the elevated diaphragm has expelled air and fluid from the pleural space through the wound opening. Hold the dressing snug until help arrives. In John's case, the doctor will insert a chest tube to prevent a tension pneumothorax.

Now, see that John stays in Fowler's position to facilitate ventilation. With penetrating wounds, you're apt to find all sorts of foreign material — bits of clothing, automobile parts, bullets or other missiles — embedded in the chest. John, for example, may have clothing or wood splinters in his wound, but don't waste time searching for them or trying to remove them — not until he's breathing adequately.

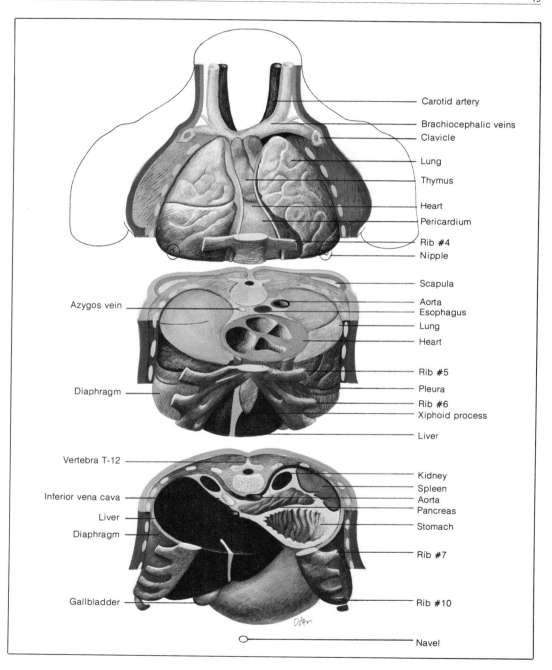

Carotid artery
Brachiocephalic veins
Clavicle
Lung
Thymus
Heart
Pericardium
Rib #4
Nipple

Scapula
Aorta
Esophagus
Lung
Heart
Rib #5
Pleura
Rib #6
Xiphoid process
Liver

Azygos vein
Diaphragm

Vertebra T-12
Inferior vena cava
Liver
Diaphragm
Gallblader

Kidney
Spleen
Aorta
Pancreas
Stomach
Rib #7
Rib #10
Navel

Pressure on the heart

INCIDENCE
Cardiac tamponade results when
fluid, blood, or clots become
trapped between the heart muscle
and the pericardial sac or anterior
chest wall. Pressure builds,
hampering ventricular filling and
reducing cardiac output.
Pressure in the pulmonary and
systemic veins rises.
   Watch for signs of cardiac
tamponade in patients with
penetrating cardiac wounds.
More frequently, it develops as a
postoperative complication of
cardiac surgery.

SYMPTOMS
Look for agitation and cyanosis.
The patient insists on sitting
upright, leaning slightly forward.
His peripheral pulses may be
weak, absent, or paradoxical
(disappearing on inspiration, and
present but weak on expiration
due to changed intrathoracic
pressures). His neck veins will be
distended since his jugular veins
can't empty properly. Blood
pressure and urinary output fall,
but central venous pressure rises.
Heart sounds seem muffled and
distant.

TREATMENT
If you suspect cardiac
tamponade, tell the doctor
immediately. He'll perform a
pericardicentesis using a 16- to
18-gauge needle. The patient
should have EKG monitoring and
adequate fluid replacement.
Make sure defibrillators and
emergency drugs are on hand.

Once that's taken care of, take a moment to assess John's
condition. Try to mentally trace the path of the fence top as it
penetrated John's chest. The illustration on page 73 will show
you how. This will give you a rough idea of the nature and
severity of problems you'll face with any thoracic injury.
Caution: If an object such as a knife is protruding from the
chest when your patient arrives, leave it in place until an
attending doctor or surgical resident can estimate the depth
and direction of injury.

Penetrating trauma to the central chest — the location of
John's injury — can cause serious pulmonary injury or a
potentially fatal cardiac injury. Cardiac tamponade could result from such an injury, because blood in the unyielding
pericardial sac seriously hampers ventricular filling and causes
a life-threatening drop in cardiac output. (To treat cardiac
tamponade competently, you must first learn to recognize it.
Your intervention can be life-saving.)

Lung trauma

Does John have lung injury? Surprisingly, penetrating trauma
to the lung can be benign if no large vessel or airway has been
cut in the process. Stab wounds or bullet wounds involving
only the spongy lung tissue rarely cause massive or fatal
bleeding because vascular pressure is low. Healing generally
takes place quickly.

Look for the source of hemorrhage in John's chest wound.
Do this by assessing the nature of the blood loss. Pulmonary
blood is dark and the flow is usually nonpulsatile (although
expiratory grunting can impart a pulsatile quality to the bleeding). However, arterial blood is bright red and the flow is
pulsatile.

Although a conservative approach to lung trauma is jus-
tified, the integrity of the chest wall must be immediately
reestablished. Interstitial and intrapleural hemorrhage must be
differentiated and promptly treated with needle aspiration or
the insertion of a chest tube. As a rule, surgery will be required
if intrapleural effusion recurs; or if pleurocutaneous bleeding
can't be controlled, or if massive air leaks occur because of
bronchial rupture. Surgery is also necessary if there is laceration of the main hilar blood vessels.

Blunt trauma can also cause interstitial hemorrhage and
edema, along with actual pulmonary lacerations and even

bronchiolar rupture. Bronchiolar rupture may be overlooked until much later, when it manifests itself as persistent atelectasis. As with penetrating injuries, you should concentrate your efforts on establishing an open airway and assessing the integrity of the chest wall and effectiveness of ventilation.

Rib fractures

Even before X-rays give conclusive proof, watch for signs that John may have one or more broken ribs. For example, is he splinting or do you see swelling or feel crepitation over his rib cage? You may even *feel* the fractured bone, in some cases.

A rib usually fractures at the point of maximum applied force. But when the force is insufficient to fracture it there, the fracture occurs posteriorly where the rib is weakest. In most cases, the force is applied in an anterior-posterior direction — produced, for example, by the impact of the steering wheel against a person's chest during rapid deceleration. Ordinarily, the doctor will treat the major symptoms — pain and instability — with local anesthetics and, later, nonnarcotic analgesics, but not restrictive bandaging.

John could have a flail chest if four or more of his ribs are fractured, or if he has a fracture of the sternum at the rib junction, destroying the structural integrity of the chest wall.

Pneumothorax, hemothorax

When air leaks from a lung or bronchus punctured by a fractured rib, it can reduce the pressure gradient in the intrapleural space just as effectively as any penetrating wound. In a patient with an intact chest wall, suspect pneumothorax if you notice any asymmetrical chest movement, especially with respiratory distress. (The same may be said for hemothorax.) Other clues: swelling and palpable crepitations around the neck caused by air that has dissected upward after an injury to the apex of the lung. On auscultation, you won't hear any breath sounds over the collapsed lung or lobe, but on percussion you'll notice hyperresonance. (With hemothorax, percussion produces a dull sound.)

No matter how they're caused, pneumothorax or hemothorax can be definitively diagnosed by chest X-ray and thoracentesis. In fact, simple aspiration by thoracentesis may be the only treatment required if the air leak is small or the bleeding is minimal. More commonly, it's large and requires

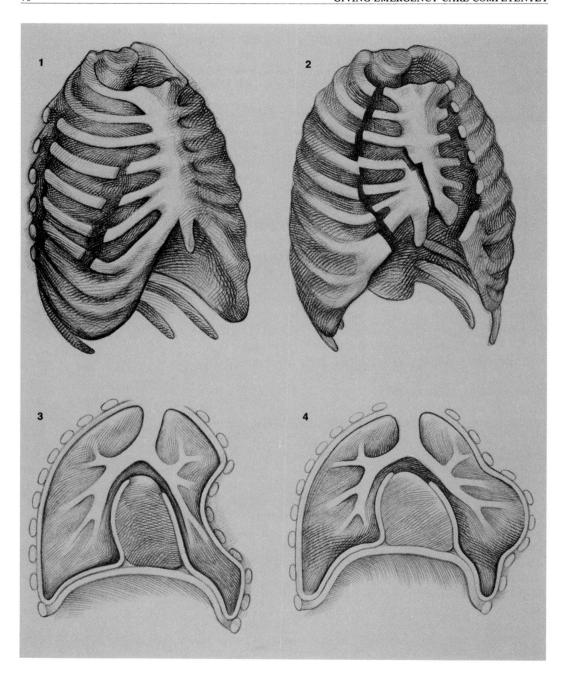

chest tube insertion and a water-seal drainage system with suction. With a minor injury, use simple gravity drainage to allow the air or blood to escape and the lung to reexpand. With more severe pneumothorax, you'll probably need suction to remove the air. John, as we mentioned before, has a chest tube. So to prevent him from developing problems, use these precautions:

• Tape all connections firmly to prevent accidental disconnection while the patient is being moved.

• Never clamp a chest tube without the doctor's specific order, unless the tube gets accidentally disconnected.

• Observe and record amount and type of drainage.

• Make sure tubing is patent and not kinked or curled.

If a major air leak occurs while the chest wall remains intact, or if chest tubes are clogged or clamped for more than a few minutes, large amounts of air can accumulate and push the mediastinum toward the unaffected lung (tension pneumothorax).

This mediastinal shift displaces the heart and great vessels, causing displacement of the point of maximum impulse (PMI) and precipitating tachycardias and arrhythmias. Of more immediate importance, the air buildup interferes with the previously unaffected lung, causing severe respiratory distress, air hunger, agitation and, eventually, cyanosis. The treatment consists of immediately inserting a chest tube — or an 18-gauge needle — to allow escape of the accumulated air. If, for some reason, a previously inserted chest tube has been clamped, then by all means unclamp it and notify the doctor.

Trauma to arteries, esophagus, or diaphragm

You won't often see laceration of large blood vessels in the neck, the superior mediastinum, or even the thorax, but when you do, realize the patient is in grave danger of exsanguination. If the laceration occurs in any cervical vessel, do the following:

• Control bleeding by direct pressure. At the same time, maintain an open airway by tracheal intubation.

• Alert the O.R. that the patient will need immediate surgery.

• Keep checking the patient's circulation and watch for motor or sensory impairment of the upper extremities.

• If the vessel is a large one, help the doctor do a cutdown in

Flail chest
Here are two kinds of flail chest, a fracture in two places of several adjacent ribs (Figure 1) and a depression of the anterior chest wall (Figure 2). Patients can sustain rib fractures without suffering breathing impairment as long as their chest wall remains stable. When fractures occur in two or more places, however, the normal rib excursion is lost. If flail chest goes untreated, the patient will quickly suffocate.

As the patient with a flail chest inspires, the chest wall over the flail area is drawn in (Figure 3); when he expires, the flail chest wall bulges out (Figure 4). In each case the flail section moves in a direction opposite to the rest of the chest wall. Because of this paradoxical motion, the lung capacity is reduced and the lung lying under the flail section can't draw in or expel air effectively.

one of the patient's lower extremities and start an I.V. of lactated Ringer's solution to replace lost fluids.

Caution: Never probe a wound of this type in the E.D.

Prompt surgery is the only treatment for transection of the aorta, an injury that may result from an automobile crash. This violent impact halts the patient's forward motion. The descending aorta swings forward, tearing the intima and media, leaving only adventitia for support. X-ray evidence of mediastinal widening and a difference in blood pressure between the arms suggest transection of the aorta; angiography confirms it.

Rule out esophageal injury in patients with multiple thoracic trauma. Check for an intact esophagus. This may require cautious passage of an indwelling aspirating tube or X-ray visualization. If you find a rupture, it'll require surgery.

The diaphragm also can be ruptured; a serious injury that may go unsuspected for long periods. Rupture of the pericardium presents signs similar to rupture of the diaphragm. This unusual event causes injury to the phrenic nerve, paralyzing the diaphragm. The resulting ventilatory insufficiency must be distinguished not only from ruptured diaphragm but also from airway obstruction. To avoid misdiagnosis, the initial evaluation should include an upright chest film and fluoroscopy. Obviously, initial management of diaphragmatic paralysis relies on respiratory support.

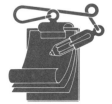

Remember these important points when caring for a patient with chest trauma:
1. Always take quick action following these priorities: establish an airway; control hemorrhage; and watch for and treat cardiac tamponade.
2. Use your ears as well as your eyes when assessing a chest wound.
3. Be alert for signs of rib fractures, such as swelling or crepitation over the rib cage.
4. Suspect pneumothorax if you notice asymmetrical chest movement, especially with respiratory distress, as well as swelling and palpable crepitation around the neck.
5. Prepare a patient with lung trauma for surgery if: intrapleural effusion recurs; pleurocutaneous bleeding can't be controlled; or massive air leaks occur because of bronchial rupture.

SKILLCHECK

1. At age 55, Guy Sloane had successful open heart surgery for aortic valve disease. His recovery seemed complete until one evening about 11 months later, when he began experiencing severe shortness of breath. His teenage daughter, who was the only person home with him at the time, called the ambulance immediately and Mr. Sloane was rushed to the hospital. By the time you see him in the emergency department, Mr. Sloane is gasping for breath; has cool, clammy skin; and looks cyanotic. His respirations sound bubbly, with moist rales over both lungs. You see frothy, blood-tinged sputum oozing from the corners of his mouth. What do you do?

2. Ten-year-old Jeffrey Wilson fell from his bicycle when he swerved to miss a dog and ran into a tree. He was unconscious when a neighbor brought him into the emergency department, though he did show signs of purposeful withdrawal when you tested him with painful stimuli. Suddenly, his breathing becomes labored, his lips and nail beds turn blue, and he starts to perspire heavily. What do you do?

3. You're just completing your 8-hour shift as triage nurse in the emergency department when Grace Swift is admitted with severe shortness of breath. She has a history of asthma, so you immediately place her in semi-Fowler's position and call the doctor. Then you administer 24% oxygen by Venturi mask to help her breathe more easily. Considering Mrs. Swift's extreme difficulty breathing, why don't you give her a higher percentage of oxygen?

4. Christine Shockley, a 39-year-old exotic dancer, is rushed to the hospital with a stab wound in her upper right chest. Her assailant withdrew the knife right after he stabbed her, so Ms. Shockley's injury is a sucking wound that can lead to complete respiratory failure. Working quickly, you take her vital signs. Her blood pressure is 80/50, her pulse rate is 126, and her respiratory rate is 32. What do you do first to keep Ms.

Shockley's breathing difficulties from getting worse?

5. Frannie Tighe is a 57-year-old housewife who only weighs 110 pounds. For years, she's suffered from allergic asthma and has been hospitalized several times when her condition has become acute. However, when you see her in the emergency department this time, her attack seems much worse. It doesn't respond to the usual therapy, and Mrs. Tighe becomes increasingly frightened. What do you do?

6. On his way home from a party, 25-year-old Joe Delnicki drove his car through a guard rail and crashed at the foot of a steep embankment. Fortunately, a passing motorist saw the accident and called the police. In less than an hour, Mr. Delnicki was extricated from the wreckage and rushed to the hospital. When you see him, he's fully conscious with multiple lacerations and puncture wounds over his entire body. You put him in Fowler's position to help him breathe easier. What do you do about the bits of clothing, dirt, and wood splinters embedded in his chest?

7. Seventeen-year-old Neil Erwin has worked hard to earn his place as quarterback on the high school football team. One afternoon, he gets injured during practice and is rushed to the hospital by the anxious football coach. When you examine Neil to determine if he needs immediate treatment, you note that he's having difficulty breathing, complains of severe pain in his left upper chest, and has swelling in that area. You feel crepitation over his rib cage. What does this tell you?

8. Two days ago, 48-year-old Sarah Espenshade underwent chest surgery for lung cancer. As he closed her wound, the doctor inserted a chest tube and attached it to a water-seal drainage bottle. Now Sarah has returned to her room and is resting comfortably. Since you're assigned to care for her, what precautions would you use to prevent problems with the chest tube?

(Answers on page 183)

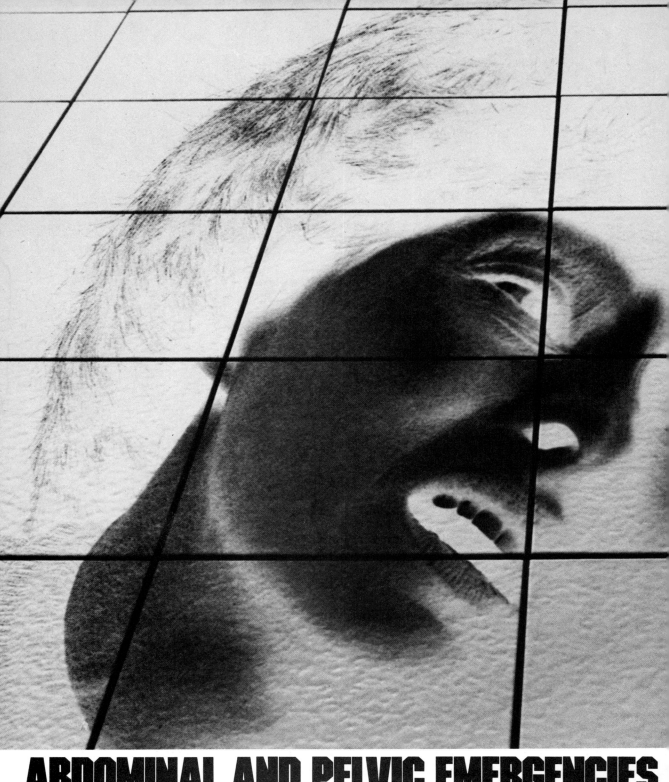

ABDOMINAL AND PELVIC EMERGENCIES

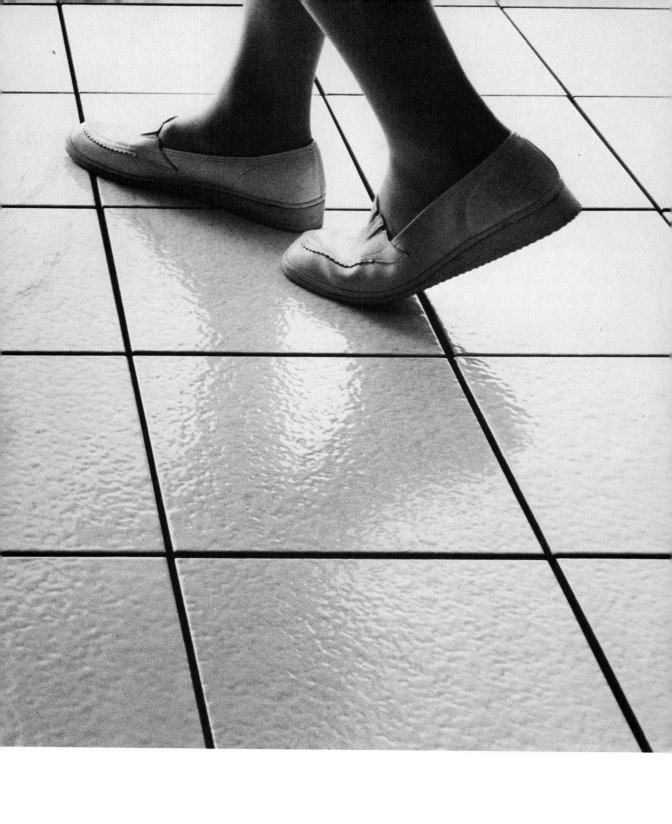

If you suspect your patient has an acute
abdominal injury, what signs and symptoms
should you look for?

What does the psoas sign indicate?

What complications occur most frequently in a
patient with a kidney injury?

What nursing actions can you take if
a pregnant patient convulses before she can
be admitted to the Ob/Gyn unit?

Can you name four care priorities when a
patient has a suspected genitourinary
emergency?

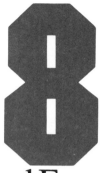

Abdominal Emergencies
How to assess the patient's pain

LOUISE MILANESE, RN, BSN

THE SCENE IN the emergency department is a tense one. Two police officers accompany the patient who's being wheeled in on a stretcher. You see immediately that he's another police officer, and note that he's pale and diaphoretic. The ambulance attendant explains that he was shot in the abdomen while attempting to stop a domestic quarrel.

Working quickly, you do a 90-second assessment of the patient's condition, as outlined in Chapter 1. The officer, whose name is Robert Teal, seems responsive and moans that the pain in his abdomen is severe and unrelenting. His blood pressure has dropped to 80/50, his pulse rate is 130, and his respiratory rate is 30.

What do you do next? Do you know what priorities to follow when you care for Officer Teal or any other patient with an acute abdomen? Do you know how to assess the patient's condition expertly so the doctor can make a quick, accurate diagnosis? What questions will he want you to ask when you take the patient's case history? What observations should you make? Which laboratory tests will the doctor need to confirm his diagnosis?

I'll give you the answers to all these questions — and many

others in this chapter. And I'll point out some nursing tips I've learned to help you work quickly and efficiently.

Recognizing an abdominal emergency

What signs and symptoms accompany an acute abdominal emergency? In many cases, you'll recognize one or more of these signs:

• severe abdominal pain, with marked tenderness on palpation; pain may or may not radiate to other parts of the body, depending on its cause

• abdominal rigidity or splinting

• nausea or vomiting; color, quantity, and consistency of vomitus may vary, depending on its cause.

Of course, you won't see all of these signs in every patient with an abdominal emergency, nor will you always see them appear in the above order. The condition causing the patient's distress determines the difference.

What are some of the conditions that can cause an acute abdomen? Officer Teal has a suspected perforation of the bowel. But a patient can develop an acute abdominal emergency because of other things: for example, severe infection, obstruction, poisoning, or rupture of an abdominal organ or blood vessel.

Whether or not the patient will need surgery to correct his condition — or diagnose it — depends on the doctor. In many cases, the patient requires *immediate* surgery to save his life.

Getting Officer Teal ready for surgery

That's the case with Officer Teal, of course. You know at once that he'll need surgery, even though you can't tell at first how severely he's been injured. So you call the doctor and alert the O.R. In most cases, he'll want you to take care of the following priorities:

• Cut away the patient's clothing, moving him as little as possible to minimize additional bleeding.

• Start an I.V. of lactated Ringer's solution. Use a large-gauge catheter so blood transfusions can be given later, if necessary.

• As you're starting the I.V., draw a blood sample for type, crossmatch, and complete blood count (CBC).

• Have a nasogastric tube inserted to aspirate the patient's stomach contents.

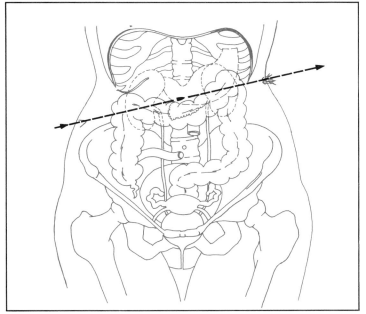

• Assist the doctor as he inserts a Foley catheter. Catheterization is necessary to measure urinary output and determine damage, if any, to the genitourinary tract.

• Reassure the patient as much as possible, and explain what he can expect. Ask if he would like to see a priest or hospital chaplain before he goes into surgery; call one, if he does.

Important: Never probe a serious abdominal wound of this type in the emergency department.

Identifying the condition

Now let's consider the conditions that give you a little more time to assess the patient — even though you must still work quickly. These conditions are cholecystitis, appendicitis, pancreatitis, and bowel obstruction.

All these bring the patient into the emergency department with severe abdominal pain, though not always of the same character and intensity. To determine which condition the patient has, the doctor relies on specific signs and symptoms. I've listed these below to help you see the differences:

• *Cholecystitis.* Sudden severe pain in right upper quadrant of abdomen, sometimes accompanied by nausea and vomit-

**Location of pain
in abdominal emergencies**

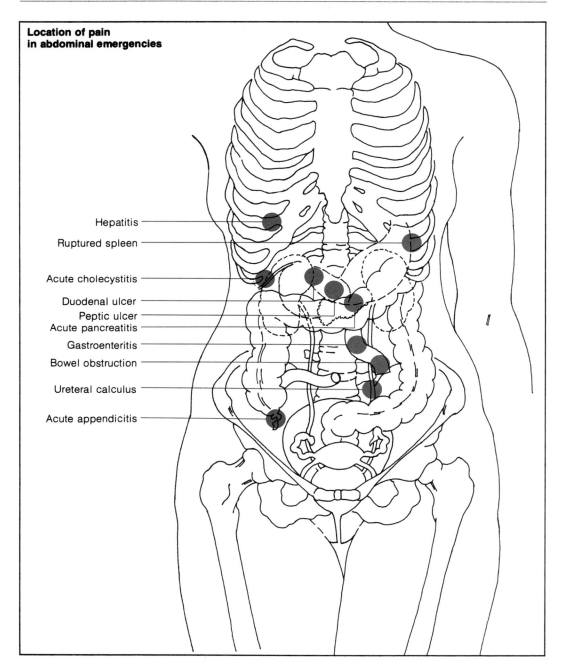

Hepatitis

Ruptured spleen

Acute cholecystitis

Duodenal ulcer

Peptic ulcer
Acute pancreatitis

Gastroenteritis

Bowel obstruction

Ureteral calculus

Acute appendicitis

ing. Pain may radiate to right scapula or shoulder, and—in many cases—may start after a heavy meal. Patient has elevated white blood count (WBC) and normal bowel sounds.

• *Appendicitis.* Mild to severe abdominal pain, generalized at first but eventually becoming localized in the right lower quadrant. Extreme tenderness and rebound soreness over appendix. Pain may be accompanied by nausea and vomiting. Patient has elevated WBC. *Caution:* Notify the doctor at once if the patient reports a sudden cessation of pain. This can indicate his appendix has ruptured.

• *Pancreatitis.* Sudden, severe pain in left upper quadrant of abdomen, sometimes accompanied by nausea and vomiting. Pain may radiate to left shoulder, and may start after heavy alcohol intake. Patient has elevated serum amylase and hypoactive bowel sounds.

• *Intestinal obstruction.* Increasingly severe abdominal pain, usually accompanied by nausea and vomiting. Patient has extremely tense, distended abdomen, and high-pitched bowel sounds. He may also have poor tissue turgor, dry mucous membranes, and feculent breath odor. Laboratory test results may show low sodium, potassium, and chloride levels; increased urine specific gravity; and slightly elevated hematocrit.

Listening and observing

As you can see, all four conditions share pain as an outstanding symptom. But there the similarity ends, and the differences in signs and symptoms begin. Part of your job is to note and record these differences, as well as any other symptoms that may suggest concurrent problems. To do this properly, you must get the patient's history—taking care to *watch* for signs that will aid the doctor in his diagnosis.

Let's talk about taking a history. What's the best way to do this when the patient's suffering severe pain and possibly nausea? Keep your questions short, and your voice calm and reassuring. Remember, the patient will probably have trouble concentrating on your questions, because his pain and vomiting (if present) will distract him. Be patient and repeat your questions, if necessary. Explain why taking a history is important.

Ask him for details about his pain. But don't use leading questions. For example, don't ask "Does your pain seem worse on your lower right side?" Just ask where it's located.

Assessing the abdomen
The drawing on the opposite page shows you where the patient will feel pain in abdominal emergencies. The more familiar you are with these emergencies and the symptoms they produce, the better nursing care you'll be able to give.

Ask him *where* the pain started, and what he was doing when it began. *Caution:* If his pain started below his mid-sternum and began after heavy exertion, it could be a myocardial infarction.

Ask him how long he's had the pain. Has he ever had anything like it before? How does it differ from previous pains in his abdomen? In what ways is it similar? Has he had any change in bowel habits? Have his stools changed in appearance? Does he have scars from previous surgery? Make sure he answers these questions thoughtfully. Sometimes a patient assumes he's having a recurrence of some previous condition (for example, gastroenteritis), when he's really suffering from something different (for example, appendicitis).

Watch the patient while you're talking to him. Does he seem to want to lie still? This suggests that his pain originates in the peritoneum rather than the thorax. The same is true if his pain gets worse when he raises his head off the pillow. Take note of these findings, so you can report them to the doctor.

Remember that a patient with abdominal pain tries to find a position that won't aggravate it. For example, a patient with appendicitis may flex his right leg to decrease pressure over the psoas muscle.

However, positioning can't be left entirely up to the patient. You must see that it's correct for his condition. Suppose the patient keeps vomiting, for instance; you'd elevate the head of his bed to prevent aspiration. *Caution:* If the patient's breathing is labored and it doesn't improve when you elevate his bed, tell the doctor at once. He may want to give the patient oxygen.

Look, listen, and palpate

As soon as you get the patient's history, examine his abdomen. Start by looking at it closely for signs that will aid the doctor in his diagnosis:

• Is the abdomen rigid or distended? Does the distention involve the entire abdomen or just a part of it?

• Do you see any obvious pulsations? Excess pulsation spreading only in an anterior direction can indicate a tumor over the aorta.

• Do you see peristaltic waves? Normally, these aren't visible. If you see waves rippling across the patient's abdomen, it can indicate intestinal obstruction.

• Is there a bluish discoloration — Cullen's sign — around

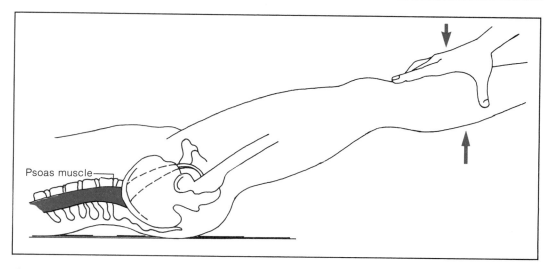

Psoas muscle

the umbilicus? This suggests an abdominal hemorrhage.

Now auscultate the patient's abdomen. Always complete this step before you begin percussion and palpation. These last two steps disturb normal abdominal sounds, hampering evaluation. Listen for peristaltic sounds; a high-pitched sound or periods of hypermotility followed by silence suggests an intestinal obstruction. Decreased peristaltic sounds (about 1 per minute) indicate paralytic ileus. Record your findings carefully and report them to the doctor.

Now palpate the patient's abdomen, covering each quadrant thoroughly. Always make sure your hands are warm before you start, and tell the patient what you're going to do. Palpate gently, because deep palpation may cause further injury. Note how much pressure the patient can tolerate on each side by watching his facial expressions and physical reactions.

Check carefully for masses; you may be able to feel a tumor or intestinal obstruction if it's large enough. Record exactly where you located it, so you can tell the doctor.

Nursing tip: If the patient has already told you which area is the most painful, leave that area till last. Then palpate it very gently, checking at the same time for rebound tenderness.

For a complete explanation of how to observe, auscultate, and palpate a patient's abdomen, read the *Nursing Skillbook* ASSESSING VITAL FUNCTIONS ACCURATELY.

The psoas sign
Have the patient lie in bed flat on his back and straighten his legs. Then ask him to raise either leg as you push down on his shin with your hand. Does this maneuver cause him pain? If it does, he most likely has an inflammation such as appendicitis near or involving the psoas muscle. Report your findings to the doctor.

The need for further findings

Naturally, everything you've done so far will help the doctor determine what's wrong with the patient. But he'll probably need further tests—as you can see on page 87—to confirm his diagnosis. So get a blood sample for CBC and differential, serum amylase, blood urea nitrogen (BUN), electrolytes, type and crossmatch. Ask the patient to void so you can get a urine sample; if he can't, you may have to catheterize him.

The doctor may want to analyze the patient's stomach contents before diagnosis—especially if the patient has been vomiting. He'll probably want a nasogastric tube inserted to completely empty the patient's stomach and small intestine.

However, make sure the tube is positioned properly before you begin irrigation. To check this, follow these guidelines:
• Aspirate a small amount of material from the tube to determine if it came from the stomach. Always check further before you assume the tube is in the stomach, though. The patient may have aspirated vomitus into his lungs.
• Instill a small amount (30 ml) of air and auscultate the patient's abdomen to determine the tube's location. Listen for a gurgling sound.
• Put the end of the tube in a pan of water. If bubbles appear, you've probably inserted the tube in a lung. Remove it at once and try again. When you're sure the tube is properly positioned, instill 30 ml of normal saline solution and aspirate a like amount of gastric contents. Make sure the tube stays patent and the suction equipment is working properly. Measure the patient's abdomen—don't just look at it—to record any change in distention.

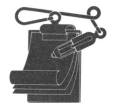

Remember these important points when caring for a patient with an abdominal emergency:
1. Be calm and reassuring when taking his history. Keep your questions short, but ask for specific details about the pain.
2. Suspect an acute abdominal emergency when a patient has severe abdominal pain with marked tenderness on palpation, abdominal rigidity or splinting, and nausea or vomiting.
3. To prepare for abdominal surgery, remove or cut away his clothing, start an I.V., draw a blood sample, and insert a nasogastric tube and a Foley catheter. Reassure patient as much as possible.

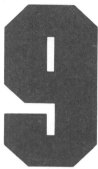

Obstetric and Gynecologic Emergencies
When fast action can save two lives

JOY P. CLAUSEN, PhD, FAAN

TODAY MARKS YOUR third day on the job in a small Ob/Gyn clinic. You've just finished taking a patient to an examination room, when 27-year-old Jodie Barr phones and asks for the doctor.

She says she's suffering severe pain in her left lower abdomen, is bleeding slightly from the vagina, and feels dizzy and weak. You ask if she's pregnant, and she replies: ''I may be. I haven't had a regular period for the past 2 months.''

Ms. Barr requires immediate emergency care in the hospital, of course. But do you know what that care would be? What condition do her symptoms suggest? What dangerous complications may occur?

You'll find out later when I get back to Ms. Barr—just one of the serious antepartum and gynecological emergencies I'll review in this chapter. Skilled nursing is a must for each of these emergencies. The care you give in the first few hours may determine whether the patient and her fetus live or die.

Abnormal vaginal bleeding: Always a danger sign
Naturally, you must recognize a condition as an emergency

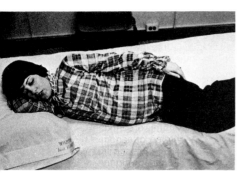

A turn for the better
In the last trimester of pregnancy and during labor, a patient lying flat on her back may suddenly become lightheaded and anxious. Although she's not bleeding vaginally, you'll find a decrease in her blood pressure and an increase in her pulse. These signs indicate supine hypotensive syndrome, caused by the gravid uterus compressing the inferior vena cava. You can easily relieve the patient's symptoms by moving her onto her side to stop the compression.

before you can treat it. And that takes knowledge and the ability to assess a patient's signs and symptoms accurately. Each condition has unique characteristics that distinguish it from conditions that are less urgent.

However, one symptom shows up in all of the antepartum emergencies I'll review, except toxemia: vaginal bleeding. Always interpret abnormal vaginal bleeding as a danger sign, because if it becomes more severe, the patient can go into hypovolemic shock.

Treating spontaneous abortions

Coping with hemorrhage and preventing shock may not be easy, even when the patient's condition is diagnosed quickly. Some antepartum emergencies pose a serious risk: for example, spontaneous abortion.

You can divide spontaneous abortions into five main groups:

• *Threatened abortion.* Pregnancy is jeopardized, but may continue. No cervical dilation present, but patient usually has bright red vaginal bleeding, mild cramps, and a slight backache.

• *Incomplete, inevitable abortion.* Products of conception partially expelled, though—in many cases—placenta remains in utero. Cervix dilated. Patient has profuse, bright red vaginal bleeding; decreased blood pressure; and, in some cases, an increased pulse.

• *Complete abortion.* Entire products of conception expelled. Cervix dilated. Patient has moderate amount of vaginal bleeding.

• *Habitual abortion.* When a woman aborts three or more times times sequentially, doctors classify her abortions as habitual. This is probably due to faulty intrauterine environment.

• *Missed abortion.* Fetus dies. Condition may not be diagnosed for several weeks or more. Little, if any, vaginal bleeding, but patient may show signs of infection: low-grade fever, pain or tenderness on examination or during sexual intercourse, and purulent vaginal discharge.

How can you help a patient who comes to the E.D. in some state of spontaneous abortion? Your main concern, as I said, is to prevent hypovolemic shock, which remains a big risk as long as the patient hemorrhages.

To illustrate, imagine your next patient is Lucille Skemp, a 23-year-old photographer's assistant who's rushed to the E.D. with an incomplete abortion. She's bleeding heavily, has cool and clammy skin, and seems extremely anxious about her condition. You take her blood pressure and find that it's 86/40. Her pulse rate is 120—and thready.

What next? Call the doctor immediately. Then take care of the following priorities as quickly as possible:

• Place patient in Trendelenburg position.

• Start an I.V. with the appropriate solution.

• At the same time you're starting the I.V., have a blood sample drawn for type, crossmatch, complete blood count (CBC), and electrolyte determination.

• Take and record vital signs every 5 minutes.

• Obtain a patient history.

Let's consider that patient history. What questions must you ask a patient like Ms. Skemp? And how can you word the questions so you won't increase her anxiety?

Start by using the term "miscarriage" when you talk to Ms. Skemp and her sexual mate—if he's there. The term "abortion" may have an unpleasant connotation for them, depending on their background and education. And you shouldn't risk upsetting them needlessly.

Find out when her bleeding started. Ask what she was doing when it began. Did she expel any clots or tissue? If she did—and didn't bring this material with her—what did it look like?

Keep track of the number of pads she uses while in the E.D. and the length of time it takes to saturate them. Save any large clots or tissue for the doctor to inspect.

Be sure to tell Ms. Skemp and her mate that she may need a dilatation and curettage, so they'll be prepared, and explain this surgical procedure. Reassure them by speaking slowly and calmly. Remember, Ms. Skemp and her mate are probably very frightened and upset.

Ask her if she's ever had a miscarriage before. If her abortions are habitual, she may have something wrong with her uterus and/or endocrine/hormonal system. To determine this, the doctor will need to do a complete examination, as well as take a complete medical history.

Note: Be sure Ms. Skemp doesn't receive an enema or a rectal or vaginal exam while waiting for the doctor. It may

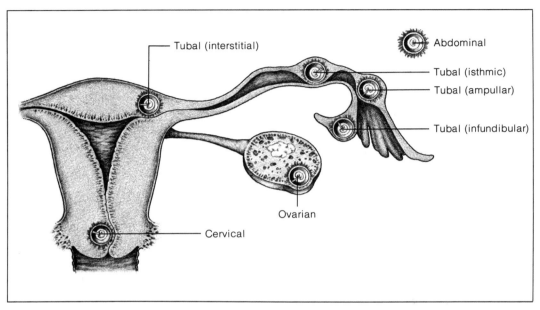

Tubal (interstitial)

Abdominal

Tubal (isthmic)

Tubal (ampullar)

Tubal (infundibular)

Ovarian

Cervical

Common sites of ectopic pregnancies
The drawing above shows where a pregnancy can develop outside the uterus. The symptoms of ectopic pregnancy may resemble those of other conditions. For a handy list that will help you tell the difference between three of the most serious gynecological disorders, see the opposite page.

increase the hemorrhaging. Also remind her—and her mate—that she can't have anything to eat or drink because she may need surgery.

Suppose the case is a threatened abortion? What can you do to help the patient? First, put her in a quiet area to keep her from becoming even more anxious. Take and record her vital signs. Be positive and reassuring.

Then, as she calms down, proceed as you did with Ms. Skemp and get a case history. Ask her how long she's been bleeding, what she was doing when it started, and how many pads she used before she came to the hospital. Record the number of pads she uses in the E.D., and save any clots or tissue she expels for examination by the doctor.

Caution: No one should give an enema to or perform a vaginal or rectal exam on a patient with a threatened abortion.

Jodie Barr: The case of an ectopic pregnancy
You'll recall Ms. Barr from the beginning of this chapter. She was rushed to the hospital with severe pain in her left lower abdomen. She was also bleeding slightly from the vagina, and felt dizzy and weak.

Now Ms. Barr arrives in the E.D., where the staff has been

alerted for a possible ectopic pregnancy. If you were the first nurse to examine her, what would you do?

First, recall what an ectopic pregnancy is: one that develops outside the uterus. Possible sites include the fallopian tubes, ovaries, cervix, abdominal cavity, or abdominal wall. Until about the 6th to 8th week of gestation, the pregnancy seems like any other. Then the fetus becomes too large for the space it's in and eventually may cause a life-threatening rupture.

Take the patient's vital signs when you suspect an ectopic pregnancy. Then call the doctor immediately. With an ectopic pregnancy, the temperature will be normal or low, unless there's been a rupture with a subsequent abdominal infection. Decreased blood pressure and increased pulse indicate internal bleeding.

Take a patient history, so the doctor can rule out other possible causes of pain. Ask the patient these questions: "How long have you had this pain. What were you doing when it started? Is there any possibility that you're pregnant? If so, for how long? Have you ever had any gynecologic problems that have caused pain? What were they? Was the pain like this?"

Have the patient point to the area where she feels the pain. Is it on only one side of her abdomen? Pain from an ectopic pregnancy or ovarian cyst is usually unilateral, though it may involve the whole abdomen. *Caution:* Get help quickly if the patient complains of shoulder-strap pain (Kehr's sign). This may mean the fertilized ovum or cyst has ruptured and she's bleeding internally.

Reassure the patient and prepare her for the possibility of surgery. Continue to monitor her vital signs closely, so that you can take steps to combat shock in case of rupture. *Important:* Never permit anyone to administer an enema or perform a vaginal or rectal exam on a patient with a possible ectopic pregnancy.

Placenta previa and abruptio placentae

Two other conditions require emergency treatment: placenta previa and abruptio placentae (see page 96). These occur primarily in the third trimester of pregnancy and are treated in the Ob/Gyn unit.

Both conditions cause significant bleeding, though they display different symptoms. For example, a patient who comes in

Symptoms of gynecological disorders

ECTOPIC PREGNANCY — uterine bleeding, spotting, cramping, abdominal pain, fainting. Gradual hemorrhaging will produce pain and pressure; rapid hemorrhaging can lead to hypotension and shock. Fever is present in late stages. During a pelvic exam, the doctor will be able to palpate an enlarged uterus and a tender mass in one fornix. The cervix will be tender to motion.

OVARIAN CYST — no striking systemic symptoms. Pelvic pain ranges from dull to intense if the ovary ruptures suddenly. The doctor will feel a palpable mass in the ovary.

PELVIC INFLAMMATORY DISEASE (P.I.D.) — severe lower abdominal pain and tenderness; fever, leukocytosis and purulent vaginal discharge, which distinguish this condition from ectopic pregnancy. When the doctor moves the cervix or palpates the adnexa during a pelvic exam, the patient will experience pain.

Placenta previa

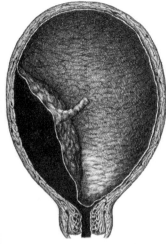

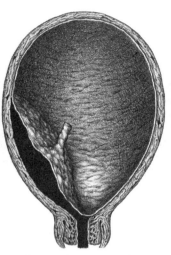

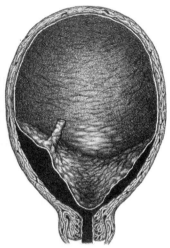

Low marginal implantation–
A small edge of the placenta
can be felt through the
internal os

Partial placenta previa –
Placenta partially caps the
internal os

Total placenta previa –
The internal os is covered
entirely

Abruptio placentae

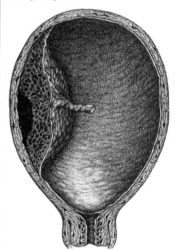

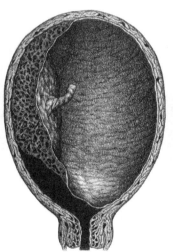

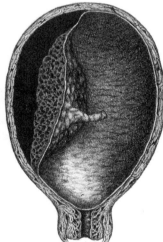

Partial separation with bleeding
between placenta and uterine
wall

Partial separation with
hemorrhage through vagina

Complete separation with
hemorrhage between placenta
and uterine wall

with placenta previa will have painless vaginal bleeding—the amount depending on the position of the abnormally implanted placenta. If the bleeding persists or an examination reveals that the placenta completely obstructs the cervical os, the doctor may perform a cesarean section, depending on gestation. If bleeding subsides, the patient will probably be treated with complete bedrest.

Consider the patient who comes in with abruptio placentae, however. Her condition is usually a more immediate emergency. She's suffering severe pain, because the placenta has dislodged from the uterine wall. She may be hemorrhaging through her vagina or inside her abdomen. The doctor will have to deliver the fetus by cesarean section or by normal vaginal delivery, depending on labor's progress.

With either of these conditions, follow the emergency care guidelines I've outlined in the section on spontaneous abortions. Prepare the patient for surgery, if needed, and do your best to reassure her. Record fetal heart rate, regularity, and strength. Remember to keep track of the number of pads she uses so you can determine blood loss, and watch for signs of developing shock. Never permit anyone to give the patient a vaginal or rectal exam, or administer an enema. Notify the nursery that the obstetrician may deliver a high-risk baby.

Toxemia: Third-ranking killer
I want to mention one other emergency condition associated with pregnancy: toxemia. This disorder, most common in the third trimester, ranks third as a cause of death among pregnant women and occurs in about 1 of every 15 pregnancies.

Toxemia can be divided into two stages—preeclampsia and eclampsia. Each presents this triad of symptoms, usually in this order: hypertension, edema, and proteinuria.

Eclampsia is the most severe form in which all symptoms are present. In addition, the patient has convulsions. Consider it an extreme emergency. The patient will need prompt—and skillful—care to protect her from injury.

If a pregnant woman convulses before she can be admitted to the Ob/Gyn unit, follow these guidelines:
• Place her securely on a flat surface.
• If possible, put a wadded-up handkerchief or washcloth part of the way into her mouth (on top of her tongue) to prevent gagging and possible airway occlusion. Take care not to

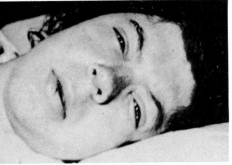

The presence of preeclampsia
The face above shows some of the classic symptoms of preeclampsia, edema of the face and eyelids and a coarsening of the features.

   To confirm suspected edema, ask the patient if her shoes or rings have become tight. And since preeclampsia can afflict a patient suddenly, teach her what symptoms to watch for between office visits. The following symptoms signal danger and should be reported to the doctor immediately: a severe frontal headache, edema of the face and hands, vision difficulties, repeated vomiting, oliguria, and epigastric pain.

injure her mouth, and if difficulty arises, insert nothing.

• Wipe away oral secretions to prevent aspiration and turn her head to one side, if possible, to promote drainage of mucus.

• Don't restrain the patient.

• Never leave the patient alone.

When the convulsion ceases, move the patient to a room that's quiet and comfortable. Remember, her bed should have padded side rails to protect her from injury if she has further convulsions.

The doctor will want her to have complete bedrest, I.V. fluids, and careful observation made of her vital signs and the fetal heart tones. You must also record her intake and output every hour, in case of renal shutdown.

Keep an emergency toxemia tray at her bedside. This should contain all the drugs she may need: antihypertensives, sedatives, diuretics, and digitalis glycosides. Make sure you also have several oral airways in case of further convulsions. To avoid increasing the patient's anxiety, put the tongue depressor where she won't see it.

Important: Don't forget the patient's family during this emergency. They'll need your reassurance, as well as your help in understanding what has happened.

For more complete information about the emergency antihypertensive drugs used to treat preeclampsia, read the *Nursing Skillbook,* GIVING CARDIOVASCULAR DRUGS SAFELY.

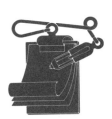

Remember these important points when caring for a patient with an obstetric/gynecologic emergency:
1. Be alert for signs and symptoms of hypovolemic shock when your patient has vaginal bleeding.
2. Use the term miscarriage to describe the condition known as spontaneous abortion when talking to a patient.
3. If the patient is bleeding vaginally, keep track of the number of pads used, and estimate the amount of drainage on each pad and the length of time it takes to saturate each one.
4. Never let anyone give an enema or perform a vaginal or rectal exam on a patient with a threatened abortion, possible ectopic pregnancy, abruptio placentae, or placenta previa.

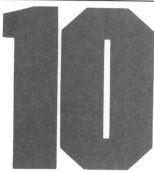

Genitourinary Emergencies
How to recognize the danger signs

LOUISE M. JULIANI, RN, MS

THE ABILITY TO MAKE a quick, accurate assessment. That's one nursing skill that tops all the rest when you're caring for a patient with an urgent genitourinary problem. How well you observe signs and symptoms — and act on them — makes a difference. It can:
- minimize pain
- keep bleeding from developing into a life-threatening hemorrhage
- prevent peritonitis
- prevent shock.

But recognizing a genitourinary emergency in time isn't the only nursing skill you'll need. Gaining the patient's cooperation when he's frightened and tense is another. Any patient who senses that something's wrong with his genitourinary tract will find it difficult — if not impossible — to relax. This creates special problems for you and the doctor treating him, especially during so necessary a procedure as catheterization.

I'll tell you how to reassure patients with serious genitourinary problems in this chapter...and also how to recognize the signs and symptoms that point to an emergency of this kind. Remember you may see one of these patients anyplace in the

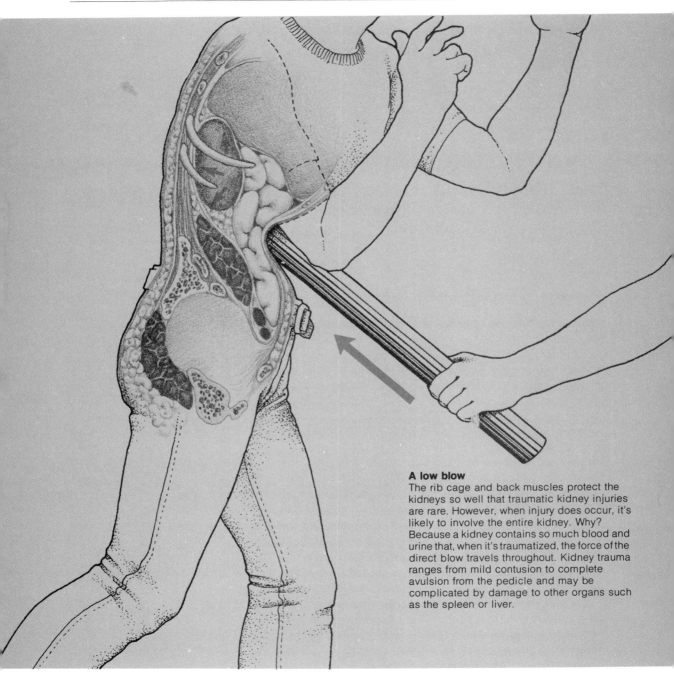

A low blow
The rib cage and back muscles protect the kidneys so well that traumatic kidney injuries are rare. However, when injury does occur, it's likely to involve the entire kidney. Why? Because a kidney contains so much blood and urine that, when it's traumatized, the force of the direct blow travels throughout. Kidney trauma ranges from mild contusion to complete avulsion from the pedicle and may be complicated by damage to other organs such as the spleen or liver.

hospital — even in the doctor's office. Urgent GU problems occur for many reasons: for example, traumatic injury to the kidney, bladder, ureter, or urethra; an obstruction or tumor; an organic disease, such as acute renal failure; or a severe fluid or electrolyte imbalance. This chapter will give you some examples to illustrate these conditions, as well as specific tips you'll find useful in caring for patients of your own.

Kidney injury: The case of a street fighter

Let's take the case of Tony Driver, a 19-year-old gang leader. You first see him at 11:30 one hot, summer night, when he's rushed to the emergency room by a police ambulance. Tony got injured in a street fight: He was struck several times in the abdomen with a two-foot section of pipe. As he's moved from the stretcher to the examination table, Tony moans that the pain's becoming worse. He gestures that it centers in his upper abdomen and radiates down his groin.

Working quickly, you and other emergency-team members assess his vital signs. But, at the same time, you try to find out as much as you can about his injury. You ask Tony to show you the exact location of the blows and to describe the pain that came immediately after. The doctor will need a urine sample to help evaluate his injuries, so if Tony can't void, prepare him for catheterization by telling him exactly what the doctor's going to do. You explain why the urine sample is needed — to check for hematuria — and ask for his cooperation. You keep reminding him that the procedure will be less painful if he's relaxed.

A traumatic kidney injury like Tony's can happen from many things: a direct blow to the upper abdomen or back; a jarring fall on the buttocks; or a penetrating wound from a bullet, knife, or sharp instrument.

Look for these telltale signs and symptoms to identify possible kidney injury:

• pain — ranging from mild tenderness on palpation to severe discomfort, even colic. Cause of pain includes injury to the kidney, renal capsule distention, and blood clots passing down the patient's ureter. Location: loin, upper abdomen, or flank, sometimes radiating down to the groin or thigh. Pain usually increases with movement.

• abdominal rigidity

• hematuria — frank or microscopic

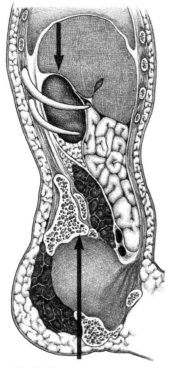

A bad fall
Falling from a height onto the buttocks causes a contrecoup injury to the kidney. The extreme force exerted on the kidney from above can tear it from the renal pedicle. The extravasation of urine into the abdominal cavity and the massive bleeding that result can kill the patient if he doesn't receive treatment rapidly.

What emergency care do you give a patient like Tony? Following the doctor's orders, use these guidelines:
- Start an I.V. of lactated Ringer's solution with a large-bore catheter, in case he'll need blood transfusions.
- Insert a Foley catheter, if necessary, to get a urine sample and to measure output. Watch for urinary retention, which may occur if blood clots block the catheter.
- Give pain medication, as ordered, when the doctor finishes his diagnostic workup. Never give it before diagnosis: A drug such as meperidine (Demerol) could mask accompanying intra-abdominal or pulmonary problems.
- Check and record vital signs frequently.
- Reassure the patient by explaining each procedure and telling him why it's needed.

Watch for these complications in a patient with kidney injury: Urinary tract hemorrhage, hypovolemic shock, and retroperitoneal bleeding. (Hypovolemic shock is discussed at length in Chapter 13.) Suspect retroperitoneal bleeding if Tony develops nausea, vomiting, or abdominal distention from paralytic ileus. When severe bleeding occurs, especially when accompanied by shock, the doctor will send the patient to the O.R.

Ureter injury: A surgical accident
Now consider the case of 56-year-old Alice Franklin, who's just returned to her room after surgery for removal of a large pelvic tumor. When you check her, you notice that she's restless and complains of pain in her right flank and right lower quadrant. You palpate her flank and discover a soft mass; then you examine the urine draining from her Foley catheter and find that it's pink. Her temperature reads 100° F. (37.8° C.).

Call the doctor immediately. Chances are, Mrs. Franklin has a damaged right ureter. The surgeon may have accidentally incised it, particularly if it was displaced by her pelvic tumor. Only rarely do ureteral injuries come from a blow or penetrating wound. Usually, they result from an abdominal or retroperitoneal surgical mishap.

Look for these telltale signs and symptoms to identify possible ureteral injury:
- pain or tenderness in flank and lower quadrant of affected side
- hematuria

- soft mass in affected flank: evidence that urine has leaked into the retroperitoneal cavity. Urine may also collect in the inguinal or suprapubic area, and in some cases, drain from the surgical wound or through the vagina.
- fever (low-grade)
- decreased urinary output. A patient probably wouldn't have anuria, unless both ureters were injured.

What emergency care do you give a patient like Mrs. Franklin? Notify the doctor at once. She'll have to return to the O.R. for reparative surgery. But don't let your actions alarm her; be calm and reassuring as you check for the signs above. Tell her you've called the doctor, who will do something to relieve her pain.

Watch for this dangerous complication in a patient with ureteral injury: peritonitis. If urine leaks into the peritoneal cavity (as it may have in Mrs. Franklin's case), you may already see some of the signs and symptoms: pain, rigid abdomen, and absent bowel sounds. Inform the doctor of your findings.

Nursing tip: Keep close watch on the urinary output of all postoperative patients, especially those who've had abdominal surgery. If a patient's output is less than 20 ml/hour for 2 consecutive hours — or you see hematuria — call the doctor immediately.

Bladder injury: When minutes count
When a patient comes in with a bladder injury, you'll see somewhat different signs and symptoms. Take the case of 32-year-old Joan Hansberry, for example, who was rushed to the hospital after being struck by a car. The doctor's already determined that she has a fractured pelvis, but she's also complaining of pain over her pubic area and has a strong urge to void. She shows signs of shock: pallor, increased pulse, and decreased blood pressure. She seems restless and appears apprehensive.

You know Ms. Hansberry's bladder may have been perforated by a fragment from her fractured pelvic bone. So you ask her to void so you can check out this possibility for the doctor. Speak calmly and confidently when you suggest voiding to her; remember she's anxious and frightened. (Patients who are tense usually have trouble voiding.)

Unfortunately, she can't void, despite her strong urge — so

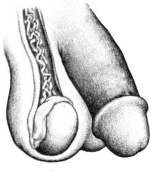

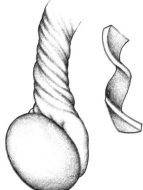

A painful twist
Torsion of the spermatic cord, an uncommon but extremely serious emergency, generally afflicts young boys. Although doctors don't know what causes this condition, they think a congenital abnormality of the tunica vaginalis or of the spermatic cord makes the scrotum red and edematous. The patient suffers severe testicular and lower abdominal pain and nausea. If the condition goes untreated for 3-4 hours, testicular ischemia can develop.

Assess the situation and call the urologist who will attempt to relieve the problem by manual detorsion. If that fails, the patient will require immediate surgery.

the doctor asks you to catheterize her. He suspects bladder injury, but he needs a urine sample to complete the diagnosis. Explain why catheterization will be necessary. Tell her how the procedure is done and emphasize that it won't cause additional pain, if she relaxes and cooperates. Remember to use strict aseptic technique and adequate lubricant when you insert the catheter. Do it gently; careless catheterization can cause infection and even further injury.

Ms. Hansberry has hematuria; this makes the doctor suspect that a bone fragment has perforated her bladder. If it had also perforated her peritoneum, she'd also run the risk of developing peritonitis. I've told you about her case to illustrate the signs and symptoms you'll see with bladder injury, and how to help the doctor evaluate them. These signs are as follows:
 • pain: lower abdominal or suprapubic area
 • evidence of shock: pallor, restlessness, apprehension, increased pulse rate, decreased blood pressure
 • strong urge to void, usually accompanied by inability to do so
 • hematuria
 • presence of a large, suprapubic mass: a perivesical collection of urine and blood.

As you know, a patient like Joan requires immediate reparative surgery.

Urethra injury: Reassuring a frightened young boy
Urethral injuries are more common in men, because of the urethra's external location. And the following case illustrates how traumatic the injury can be — and what you can do to make it less so.

Twelve-year-old Bill Abbey was riding his bike on an unfamiliar road when he hit a pothole and struck his perineum on the bike's crossbar. The injury caused Bill such intense pain that his mother rushed him to the emergency department of your hospital. A quick examination reveals a soft mass at the base of Bill's penis and blood on his external meatus.

Bill whispers that he has to urinate. But you warn him not to try. His injury may have traumatized his sphincter mechanism, making normal voiding impossible. You explain that if he does attempt to void, the urine may leak into his perineum and cause additional, painful swelling. The doctor will have to catheterize him to provide a safe outlet for the urine. Reassure Bill that the doctor knows exactly how to do this, that it's only a temporary situation, and that you will explain the procedure in detail.

You sense Bill's acute embarrassment, of course—it's almost as intense as his pain. And he's frightened, particularly by the mention of procedures that are new and unusual to him. You try to alleviate Bill's discomfort by speaking calmly and reassuringly. Tell him that other boys have suffered similar injuries and the doctor helped them.

Ask if he knows where his urethra is located and explain that it probably has a small tear in it. Be sure to answer any questions Bill may have completely and honestly. To help the tear heal, insert a Foley catheter, as ordered by the doctor.

As the you prepare to insert the rubber tip of the catheter, explain to Bill exactly what you're doing. Emphasize that you need his cooperation to get the catheter in place. Keep reminding him that he'll be "as good as new" when his injury is healed. Remember, urethral injury can traumatize a patient psychologically, as well as physically.

Those painful kidney stones
Not every genitourinary emergency starts with an injury. Many other conditions cause symptoms frightening or painful enough to bring the patient to a doctor: for example, renal calculi—or what we commonly call kidney stones.

Just having calculi in the urinary tract doesn't constitute an emergency. But when the stones cause colic, that's another matter. I'm thinking of 39-year-old Calvin White, who came to our hospital one night in severe pain. The pain woke him up, he said, and nothing he did seemed to lessen its severity.

Mrs. White reported that her husband had vomited twice on the way to the hospital. He also felt weak, cold, and bloated. We suspected renal colic, as we listened to their stories. Mr. White displayed all the classic signs and symptoms:
- severe, unremitting pain, usually confined to the kidney area. However, it may also extend to the abdomen, thigh, or genitalia.
- nausea, vomiting, and occasional abdominal distention from paralytic ileus
- hematuria. May be microscopic, but always present.

What emergency care do you give a patient like Mr. White?

First, gather information about his medical history. He may have suffered renal colic attacks before and have some idea what's happening. The doctor can't confirm his diagnosis until he gets an intravenous pyelogram (IVP) of the patient's kidneys. But he may order morphine I.M. to alleviate pain.

Be calm and reassuring. Chances are, the patient with renal colic will have to stay in the hospital, where increased fluid intake and daily exercise will help him pass the stones. Explain how he will have to strain his urine through gauze to catch any stones. If they don't pass spontaneously and pain continues, he may require surgery.

Oliguria and anuria: Two danger signs

Never ignore oliguria (diminished urinary output) or anuria (absence of urinary output) when they occur. These two symptoms require immediate attention, because they may be caused by one of the following conditions: acute or chronic renal failure; severe fluid and electrolyte imbalance; injury to urinary tract; or urinary tract obstruction.

Whenever a patient complains of either condition—or you note them on his intake/output record—notify the doctor immediately and get a complete medical history. Don't forget to ask about changes in diet, especially when the patient is elderly, diabetic, or apt to try fasting. Be alert for clues that may point to the cause of the condition: for example, fatigue; rapid weight loss or gain; or elevated serum creatinine, blood urea nitrogen, and potassium levels.

Remember these important points when caring for a patient with a genitourinary emergency:
1. Suspect a possible kidney injury in a patient with loin, upper abdomen, or flank pain, possibly radiating to groin or thigh; abdominal rigidity; and frank or microscopic hematoma.
2. Suspect a ureteral injury in a patient with pain or tenderness in flank and lower quadrant of affected side, hematuria, soft mass in affected flank, low-grade fever, and decreased urinary output.
3. To detect possible urinary tract damage, closely monitor urinary output in a patient who's experienced an abdominal injury.

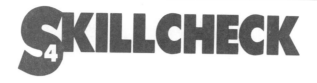

1. About two hours ago, Gertrude Bingham, a 50-year-old saleslady, returned to her room after undergoing a hysterectomy. At the time, she was alert and responsive and her vital signs were normal. When you check her now, however, her condition is changed. She seems restless and complains of pain in her right flank and right lower quadrant. When you take her temperature, you discover that it reads 100° F. (37.8° C.) The urine draining from her Foley catheter is slightly pink. What do you think is wrong?

2. Margery Vreeland, who is 25 years old and 8½ months pregnant, is rushed to the emergency department after being hurt in a car accident. She has some minor lacerations on her arms and legs, but she's mainly concerned about her fetus. Since the accident, she's begun to have mild contractions (about 5 minutes apart) and has bright red bleeding from her vagina. What do you do next?

3. Thomas Rozecki is a 29-year-old construction worker, who has been working on an apartment building project for the past year. One day, he falls off a 12-foot scaffold and lands on his buttocks. Three of his co-workers rush him to the emergency department where you are a triage nurse. How would you determine if Mr. Rozecki has possible kidney damage?

4. Shortly after breakfast one hot summer morning, 72-year-old Clare Becker is rushed to the hospital by her daughter Beatrice. About an hour before, Mrs. Becker started having crampy abdominal pains and vomited once. Now the pains have become much worse, and Mrs. Becker and her daughter are frightened. A quick examination reveals that Mrs. Becker's abdomen is rigid and distended and she has high-pitched bowel sounds. Her breath smells feculent. What does this suggest to you?

5. You've just finished admitting a patient with a fractured ankle, when 24-year-old Sylvia Gibbons — who is 5 months pregnant — is brought to the emergency department by her anxious husband. Mrs. Gibbons has heavy vaginal bleeding, cool and clammy skin, and seems extremely anxious. Her blood pressure is 86/40 and her pulse rate is 120. You suspect she's having a spontaneous abortion. What do you do?

6. You're a nurse in a doctor's office. Shortly before closing time one afternoon, you receive a phone call from 32-year-old Marie Cook, who seems to be very distressed. She says she's suffering severe pain in her right lower abdomen, is bleeding slightly from the vagina, and feels dizzy and weak. What do these symptoms suggest to you? What question do you immediately ask of Mrs. Cook?

7. You hear the ambulance pull up to the emergency department entrance, and minutes later two paramedics wheel in a middle-aged bank guard with a gunshot wound in the abdomen. He's bleeding heavily and showing signs of hypovolemic shock. His blood pressure is 80/50, his pulse rate is 130, and his respirations 30. You call the doctor immediately. What can you do to help the bank guard while you're waiting for the doctor to arrive?

(Answers on page 183)

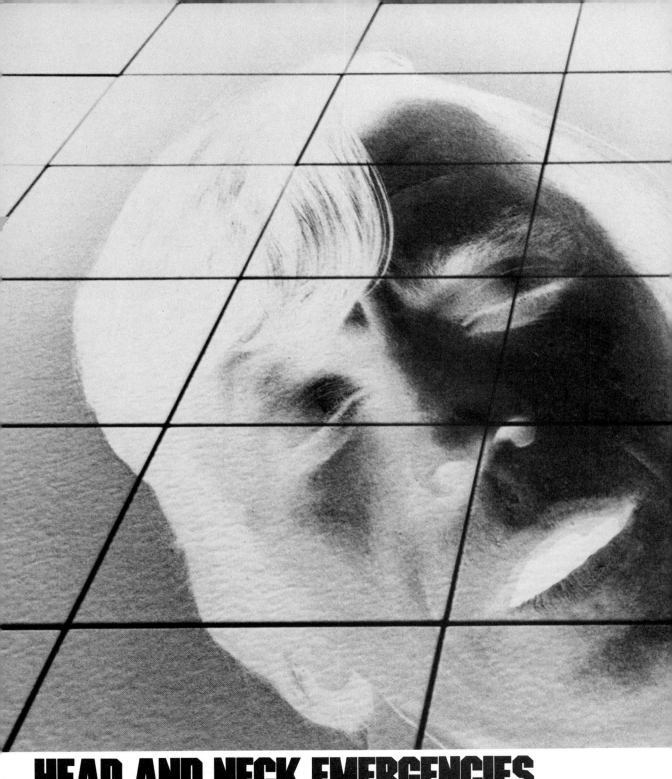

HEAD AND NECK EMERGENCIES

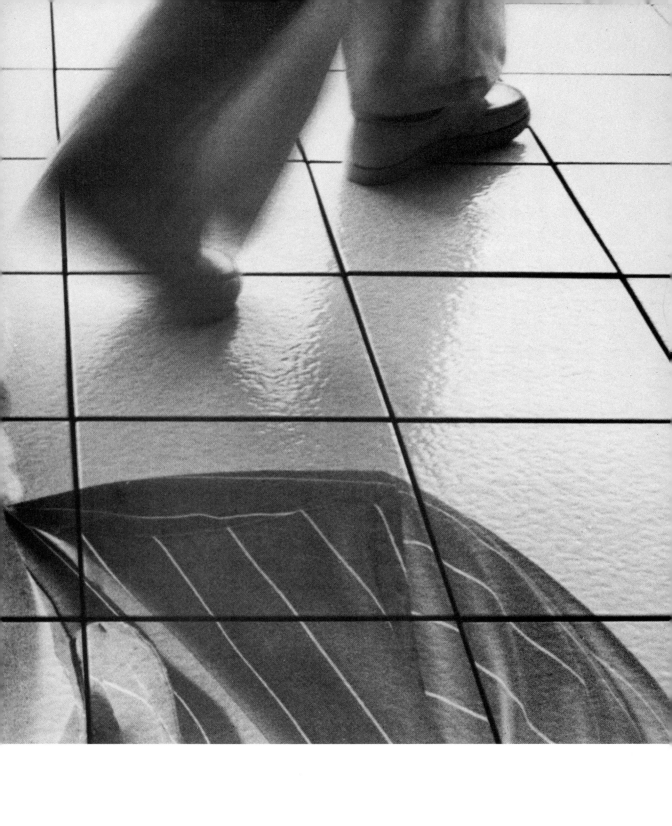

What underlying disease may cause severe, unexplained nosebleeds?

How do you help a patient with an insect in his ear?

What emergency care guidelines are indicated when a patient has a suspected fractured larynx?

Do you known the proper procedure for clearing a head-injured patient's airway?

What two types of head injuries cause the most severe brain damage?

What complications may result from a severe head injury?

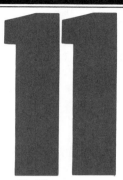

Eye, Ear, Nose, and Throat Emergencies
When life or vision is threatened

JEANNE DUPONT, RN

YOU'VE JUST COME ON DUTY when 29-year-old Bud Henry arrives in the emergency department of your hospital complaining of severe throat pain. You see at once that he's very ill; in fact, he can hardly talk or swallow. His temperature reads 104° F. (40° C.), his breathing seems labored, and he's becoming very restless. You prepare for the immediate possibility of airway obstruction — the most serious emergency you'll face when a patient has a throat problem.

Hemorrhage emergencies, of course, run a close second in patients with nose and throat problems. And these two crises require prompt and effective action on your part to save the patient's life.

In my part of this chapter, I'll talk about nose and throat problems — confining it to those that truly endanger life. You can review what to do for eye emergencies that threaten vision in a special section on page 117. And you'll learn how to help children who come in with ear, nose, and throat problems on page 116.

Two dangerous throat infections
Now, let's get back to Mr. Henry, who's suffering from a

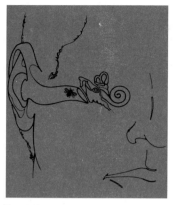

It can bug you
A person can get an insect in his ear, though it happens rarely. When it does, the noise and movement of the trapped insect can be extremely traumatic. When a patient comes to the E.D. with this emergency, assure him that you'll be able to help him quickly. Have him sit still, then instill a few drops of alcohol into the ear with the insect. The alcohol anesthetizes the insect so you can remove it with an appropriate instrument. Once the insect has been extracted, the doctor may prescribe antibiotic ear drops to prevent infection.

peritonsillar abscess. Naturally, you don't know the diagnosis until the doctor examines him, but you do know that some severe throat infections can obstruct a patient's airway. In Mr. Henry's case, the doctor finds an abscess and reports that his tonsils, uvula, and surrounding throat tissues appear swollen. Mr. Henry has only a small airway open when the doctor checks him, and—as the infection progresses—that could close at any time.

Because you're aware of this danger, you already have a tracheostomy set and suction equipment ready, and you watch him carefully. As the doctor drains the abscess, orders antibiotics, and gets Mr. Henry ready for admission to the hospital, you're alert for the following:
• change in breathing pattern
• change in respirations: rate increased; more shallow
• change in skin color: patient may show cyanosis
• change in behavior: patient may become very restless and apprehensive from anoxia.

Call these changes to the doctor's attention immediately: He may have to perform a tracheotomy. Even if Mr. Henry's airway remains open, make sure he's watched closely when he's transferred to another unit. Advise the staff to keep a trach set ready at Mr. Henry's bedside.

Epiglottitis—inflammation and edema of the epiglottis from infection—is another condition that can quickly obstruct a patient's airway. At one time, we thought it occurred only in children, but now we see it many times in adults.

The patient usually reports that he had just a sore throat at first, but it increased in severity. By the time you see him, he's having trouble breathing and may not be able to close his mouth. In most cases, he's restless (from lack of oxygen) and has a fever.

Always keep a trach set and suction equipment handy when you suspect a patient has epiglottitis and watch for the signs listed above. *Remember:* A laryngoscope exam should only be performed in the operating room by the doctor. This exam may trigger respiratory arrest and make a tracheotomy necessary.

What's stuck?
A severe throat infection isn't the only condition that can cause airway obstruction. For example, if a patient accidentally gets a

foreign body lodged in his throat, he's also in danger.

Take the case of Francis Miller, a 35-year-old violinist, who got a small piece of steak caught in his throat during a banquet. He can still breathe, but he says it hurts to swallow. He points to the exact spot where he thinks the steak is lodged, which appears to be just above his larynx.

What's your first step as the doctor prepares to examine Mr. Miller? First, have a tracheostomy set and suction equipment ready. You never know when a foreign body could shift from its original position and totally obstruct the airway. (If that happens, you might try expelling the object from the patient's airway with the abdominal thrust maneuver. For complete details on how—and when—to try this method, see Chapter 6.)

Since Mr. Miller is still breathing, though, try to prevent the piece of steak from shifting to another spot. Have him sit upright and tell him not to move.

Gain Mr. Miller's cooperation by explaining what to expect. For example, start by telling him that the doctor will spray his throat with a local anesthetic. Then ask him to stick out his tongue, so you can hold it in place with a sponge while the doctor examines his throat. If the doctor locates the steak, he'll try to remove it with curved forceps. Instruct Mr. Miller to pant like a puppy during this procedure to reduce his tendency to gag.

Mr. Miller is lucky. With your help, the doctor removes the piece of steak successfully. Chances are, the doctor couldn't have reached it if it had lodged further down in his larynx or esophagus. He'd have needed an X-ray to determine the meat's location and then he'd have sent Mr. Miller to the O.R.

Nursing tip: Remember to tell a patient like Mr. Miller not to eat or drink anything until the anesthetic effect wears off his throat. If he doesn't wait till the numbness leaves, he risks choking and aspirating food or liquid.

Rhonda: The girl with the fractured larynx

Rhonda Harrington, a 23-year-old tennis instructor, was rushed to the emergency department after an automobile accident. The doctor suspects that she has a fractured larynx, because her cervical area looks flat and he can feel no thyroid cartilage.

Rhonda has severe face and neck pain, can't speak above a whisper, and indicates that it's difficult to swallow. You note

Nose care after a nosebleed
Here are some instructions to give your patient after the doctor has stopped the patient's nosebleed.
1. Do not pick your nose or insert anything into it (such as cotton swabs, handkerchiefs, or tissues). Do not blow your nose forcefully.
2. If you must sneeze, expel the sneeze through your open mouth.
3. On the first day after your appointment, don't stoop or exert yourself physically. When you lie down, elevate your head using two or three pillows.
4. On the second day, put a little petroleum jelly just inside your nostrils to soften the crusts that form after a nosebleed. Continue this treatment for 7 days.
5. Avoid hot drinks and alcoholic beverages for 4 days.
6. Don't smoke or take aspirin for 5 days.
7. If you're constipated, take a laxative. Avoid straining.
8. If possible, use a cold-mist humidifier at night.
IF BLEEDING STARTS AGAIN:
1. Sit up with your head slightly forward, and squeeze the lower half of your nose between your thumb and index finger. Keep up this pressure for 10 minutes.
2. Sometimes a piece of moist cotton placed high inside your upper lip and in front of your upper teeth will stop the bleeding.
3. If these remedies fail, cold water or ice compresses on the outside of your nose may help.
4. If the bleeding continues, call the doctor immediately, and go to the closest hospital's emergency department for treatment.

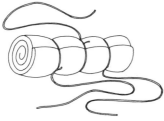

The anterior-posterior pack
1. To make a posterior pack, roll 4″ x 4″ gauze and cut to size. Secure it by tying three silk twist threads around it.
2. Assist the doctor as he inserts a #14 or a #16 French catheter into each nostril. He then grasps the catheters with a Kelly clamp and pulls them out through the mouth.
3. Attach the two lateral sutures of the pack to the catheters (Figure 1, page 115).
4. The doctor pulls the pack into place above the soft palate by withdrawing the catheters gently from the nose (Figure 2, page 115). As he pushes the pack into the nasopharynx, he'll pull the pack's strings through the nostrils.
5. You'll have to hold the sutures as tightly as possible with a Kelly clamp while the doctor inserts an anterior pack.
6. An anterior pack consists of ½″ Iodoform or ½″ Vaseline gauze lubricated with antibiotic ointment. (Sometimes an anterior pack alone will control bleeding.) The doctor will insert this carefully into the nose using bayonet forceps.
7. Tie the lateral strings securely around a dental roll to provide support and prevent irritation.
8. The doctor brings the third suture of the posterior pack out the mouth and tapes it to the cheek.
9. After this procedure the patient will be sedated and hospitalized. The packs will remain in place for 2 to 5 days.

that the skin covering her larynx feels swollen and seems like it's stretched over crumpled cellophane. You recognize this immediately as subcutaneous emphysema, a condition in which air from a crushed larynx escapes beneath the skin.

What do you remember as you give emergency care to a girl like Rhonda? Follow these guidelines, keeping them in mind whenever you see any patient with severe face and neck injuries:

• Prepare for possible airway obstruction. Have a trach set and suction equipment handy.

• Check vital signs frequently and watch the patient closely for signs of respiratory distress (see page 18).

• Never leave the patient alone.

The other killer: Hemorrhage
Now let's consider the second life-threatening emergency that can occur when a patient has a nose or throat problem: hemorrhage. You'll face it when you treat a patient with a severe nosebleed — and you may see it in a patient who has recently had a tonsillectomy.

To start, I'll explain how you care for a patient with a severe nosebleed. Your role as a nurse focuses on these responsibilities:

• Get an accurate medical history.

• Assist the doctor in whatever method he chooses to stop the bleeding.

• Gain the patient's cooperation by reassuring him and explaining in detail what needs to be done.

• Teach the patient how to prevent further nosebleeds.

Severe nosebleeds aren't just nosebleeds, as you know. They may point to an underlying disease, such as hypertension or a blood dyscrasia. Or they may be due partly to a drug the patient is taking, such as an anticoagulant. Your skill at asking the right questions will help the doctor determine how to treat the patient's nosebleed. Most nosebleeds stop when direct pressure or cautery is applied. But some require more complicated procedures, such as the anterior pack or anterior-posterior pack.

Your first step, after you call the doctor, is to reassure the patient and get his medical history. Begin by telling him to sit down with his head bent slightly forward — so the blood won't drain down his throat and cause him to choke. Then show him

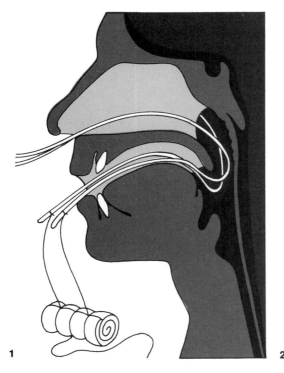

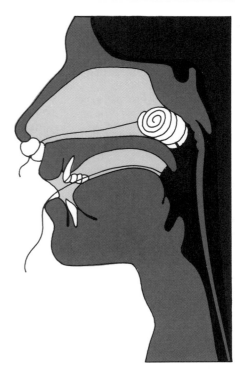

Placing posterior pack

how to squeeze the front part of his nose, near his nostrils, with a 4″ x 4″ sponge. Reassure him that he won't bleed to death by explaining that the doctor knows special ways to control bleeding.

Now, get as much information as you can from the patient. If he can't answer your questions, ask the person who accompanied him to the hospital. Ask these questions:

• Have you had any nosebleeds before and, if you have, how long ago?

• Are you being treated for any condition or disease, such as high blood pressure, heart disease, or a blood disorder?

• Are you taking any drugs; for example, a ''blood thinner'' or ''blood pressure medicine''? What dosage are you taking?

When the patient appears more relaxed, take his blood pressure and arrange to have necessary blood work done. Sometimes a patient's blood pressure is high, even though he's been taking an antihypertensive drug. If that's the case, ask how long it's been since he's had a checkup. Record the

Pediatric emergencies

FOREIGN BODY IN THE NOSE
When a child inserts an object into his nose, the foul-smelling discharge that results alarms the parents, who bring the child to the doctor.

Ask the child if he's put something up his nose. Then explain that you're going to help him. Tell the parent that an otolaryngologist will remove the object easily, if it's visible, with a nasal speculum and bayonet forceps, Fogarty catheter, or suction forceps.

Depending on the child's age, he may have to be restrained with an Olympic papoose or a blanket wrapped around him. Let the parents help you, unless they're apt to become frightened or anxious.

If the doctor can't see the foreign body in the nose, he may insert cocaine packs to anesthetize the area, shrink mucous membranes, and facilitate examination. After removal, the doctor may prescribe antibiotics.

FOREIGN BODY IN THE EAR
If a child is brought to the E.D. with an object in his ear, you'll probably have to restrain him before you can remove it. Tell the child how you're going to help him. Then use a Pedi-wrap, an Olympic papoose, or a blanket wrapped around the child to keep him still. Position his head and hold it firmly in place.

The doctor will use angled forceps or "alligator" forceps to remove the object. Or he may use a suction tip or a suction cup.

If the object is difficult to remove, the doctor will anesthetize the child first to alleviate his pain and anxiety. Antibiotic ear drops may be ordered to prevent infection.

information with your other findings and tell the doctor.

As I mentioned before, the doctor can stop most severe nosebleeds with some form of cautery. Explain the procedure to the patient so he'll cooperate and won't be so frightened. Encourage him to ask questions. Answer his questions completely and honestly. If the doctor decides to put in an anterior pack or an anterior-posterior pack, you'll have to prepare the patient thoroughly. You need to know exactly how to assist during these last two procedures. For complete details on what to do, see the captions on page 114.

Teaching the patient how to prevent further nosebleeds is your final responsibility before he leaves the hospital. Do this by giving him a list of instructions—such as the one on page 113—and discussing each point. Demonstrate how to stop bleeding, if it starts again, and make sure he understands you. Remind him to call the doctor anytime he can't stop the bleeding promptly or if he has frequent nosebleeds.

Hemorrhage after tonsillectomy

Another emergency you may see involving the throat is hemorrhage after tonsillectomy. This occurs when one or more sutures dissolve before healing is complete. I've known this type of hemorrhage to happen within the first 24 hours after surgery, but that's unusual. Generally, it occurs from 5 to 10 days after surgery, if it occurs at all.

What's the patient like? He usually arrives in the emergency department with a basin of blood in his hands, and he's pale, extremely anxious, and diaphoretic. Call the doctor immediately and watch the patient closely. He may faint, fall against something, and injure himself further.

Loss of blood may be extensive in this type of hemorrhage, so move quickly. For starters, start an I.V. with lactated Ringer's solution to keep a vein open and to prevent shock. In most cases, the doctor will probably try to stop the bleeding with cautery or an emergency tonsil suture (Ethicon Plain O Taper FN-2). If the patient is a child, keep in mind that the loss of a lot of blood quickly is much more critical than in an adult.

Keep the patient sitting up while you're waiting for the doctor. This will prevent him from choking on his blood. Remember, he's no doubt very frightened by what's happened, so be calm and reassuring. If the doctor plans to cauterize or suture the wound in the emergency department, prepare the

HOW TO CARE FOR EYE EMERGENCIES

CONJUNCTIVITIS (Figure 1). Allergy, infection, or physical or chemical trauma can cause an inflammation of the conjunctiva, which produces redness, pain, swelling, lacrimation, and possible discharge. This condition is an emergency because it frightens the patient.

If the conjunctivitis is caused by an allergy, apply cold compresses; if it's caused by an infection, however, apply warm compresses. Instill therapeutic ointment or drops, as ordered. Do not irrigate eye, unless the conjunctivitis is the result of chemical trauma.

Before he uses the medication, have the patient wash his hands and dry them with a clean towel.

GLAUCOMA. Intraocular pressure increases rapidly, causing severe pain in and around the eye.

The patient's vision becomes cloudy and blurred. He may see halos around lights. His pupils will appear fixed and mid-dilated. He may suffer nausea and vomiting. Untreated, glaucoma can cause blindness.

The doctor will prescribe drugs to reduce intraocular pressure and pain. If these don't work, he'll have to perform surgery.

Reassure the patient and explain all procedures. Have him avoid exertion or emotional upset.

RETINAL DETACHMENT, OR HORSESHOE TEAR OF THE RETINA (Figure 2). A separation of the retina from the choroid is usually associated with a hole or tear in the retina. This condition may be caused by degenerative changes, trauma from a blow, eye surgery, or diabetes.

Besides complaining of painless, blurred vision, the patient may see flashes of light, spots,

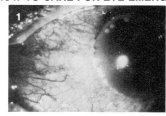

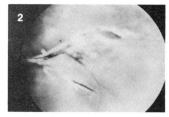

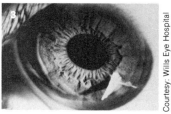

Courtesy: Wills Eye Hospital

or a veil-like covering before his eyes. Some areas of his vision may be entirely blank.

Reassure the patient, and instruct him to remain in bed. Since both his eyes may be bandaged, identify yourself when you enter the room and avoid bumping the bed.

If the patient complains of severe pain, blurred or double vision, suspect internal damage. The doctor may order laser treatments or surgery to prevent blindness. The doctor determines how the patient is positioned. If the patient's condition requires surgery, administer a sedative and prepare the patient, as ordered.

TRAUMATIC INJURIES. In all trauma cases, call the ophthalmologist.

Chemical burns: Copiously flush the lids, conjunctiva, and cornea continuously with water for at least 15 minutes. Make sure the patient lies on the affected side so you don't wash the chemical into his other eye.

Corneal abrasion: The doctor will prescribe antibiotic eye drops to prevent infection.

To further aid healing, the patient may wear a patch over his eye for 24 to 36 hours. Explain these procedures, to ease anxiety.

Foreign bodies: If an object is imbedded in the patient's cornea, as in Figure 3, call the ophthalmologist immediately; surgery may be needed.

Sometimes a patient merely has a dust particle or insect in his eye. In a case like this, have the patient look upward. As he does, evert his lower lid to expose the conjunctival sac. Gently remove the particle with a small cotton applicator dipped in saline.

If you can't find the foreign object in the lower lid, have the patient look downward so you can examine the upper lid. To do this, place a cotton applicator on the outer surface of the upper lid. Then gently hold the patient's eyelashes and pull the upper lid out and over the cotton. Use another cotton applicator moistened in saline to remove the particle.

Blows to the eye: Treat external injuries with ice to prevent edema. Have the patient continue this for 24 hours and then apply heat, as needed. If the patient complains of severe pain, or blurred or double vision, suspect internal damage. Refer the patient to an eye doctor for an examination.

patient for what will happen by explaining the procedure. Tell him that the bleeding will stop, but you need his cooperation. Warn him not to move while the doctor is working, and help by steadying his head with your hands.

Because hemorrhaging is so frightening, keep reassuring the patient as the doctor works on him. Repeating the steps of the procedure the doctor is using may ease the patient's anxiety.

Seconds count whenever hemorrhage occurs, so learn what equipment and drugs your doctor will need in advance and have them ready. Never waste precious time by not being prepared.

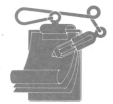

Remember these important points when caring for a patient with an eye, ear, or throat emergency:

1. Be alert for signs and symptoms of an airway obstruction in a patient with a peritonsillar abscess or epiglottitis.

2. Before removing an insect from your patient's ear, instill a few drops of alcohol into the ear to anesthetize the insect.

3. Never use the abdominal thrust manuever to remove a chicken or fish bone. Doing so may cause the patient serious injury.

4. Apply a cold compress to the eye of a patient with conjunctivitis resulting from an allergy.

5. Suspect a retinal detachment or tear in a patient complaining of blurred vision, flashes of light, or a veil-like covering before his eyes.

6. Act quickly to prevent shock in a patient with a posttonsillectomy hemorrhage.

12

Head and Spinal Injuries
How to prevent lasting neurologic damage

NANCY SWIFT-BANDINI, RN

THE BUSY HOLIDAY WEEKEND has almost ended, and you're completing the last of an 8-hour shift in the emergency department. From far away, you hear the harsh warbling of the ambulance approaching the hospital and, soon after, attendants bring in Randy Clarke, a 20-year-old college student from a nearby community. According to witnesses, Randy was thrown from his motorcycle when he swerved to miss a cow that had wandered out onto the road.

You see at once that Randy is comatose, and you suspect possible head injury. Fortunately, his respirations are adequate, but you notice a small amount of clear fluid leaking from his nose and right ear.

What next? Do you know the proper emergency care to give a patient like Randy? How would you assess his injury? Can you list the steps on a neurologic checklist? Do you know how to position a head-injured patient? Suppose you also suspect he has a spinal cord injury? Can you correctly identify a spinal fluid leak? Do you know what to do about it?

I'll answer these questions for you—as well as others you may have thought of. But first, I want to tell you more about head injuries and how they affect the brain.

Symptoms of increasing intracranial pressure

RESPONSE LEVELS:
Considerable variation:
Alert, lethargic to drowsy, or
stuporous to comatose

PULSE:
Rate slows to 60 or below, or
increases to 100 or above

RESPIRATION:
Rate slows with longer periods of
apnea; patient may have irregular
respirations and Cheyne-Stokes or
Kussmaul breathing

BLOOD PRESSURE:
Diastolic pressure falls; pulse
pressure widens

TEMPERATURE:
Rises moderately; does not
usually elevate unless extensive
brain compression is present

SKIN SURFACE TEMPERATURE:
Normal until fever develops

When a patient has suffered head injury, your primary concern isn't the condition of his skull or scalp, but the condition of his brain and the degree of damage done to it. A skull fracture by itself isn't that significant, unless it presses on the brain or is accompanied by leakage of cerebrospinal fluid. (For a description of differences in skull fractures, see page 122.)

Damage to the brain falls into two main categories, as you'll recall — concussion and contusion. Concussion, less severe of the two, happens when the brain gets jostled from a direct or indirect blow. Concussion can leave the patient dazed or unconscious, though unconsciousness may last only a few seconds or minutes. In most patients, symptoms usually disappear within 48 hours and recovery is complete.

Always consider contusion (multiple bruising of the brain) more serious than concussion. It may cause loss of consciousness so profound that the patient dies within a few hours. Or with a less severe injury, the patient may act drowsy or confused. He may even become agitated and violently reject your attempts to care for him. This period can last for days or weeks.

The rebound reaction

Now let's talk about what happens inside a person's skull when his head gets injured. A lot depends on the type of injury he receives: coup-contrecoup or acceleration-deceleration.

To illustrate: When a person falls and hits his head on a hard object — or gets hit with a baseball bat — he receives a coup-contrecoup injury. The blow bruises his brain just beneath the site of the trauma as the skull rebounds against it. Then, as the transmitted blow drives the full force of the brain's weight to the opposite side of the head, contrecoup injury may follow. Additional hemorrhages may occur where the brain strikes the bony prominences of the skull, such as the sphenoidal ridges. Contusions with lacerations of the brain's blood vessels can produce considerable blood loss. Blood then collects beneath the dura mater, forming a subdural hematoma.

I can best illustrate an acceleration-deceleration injury by asking you to imagine a person whose car skids off the road and hits a tree. His head gets hurled forward, then snaps backward as the car comes to a halt. Inside the skull, his brain rebounds against bony ridges and may be bruised and lacer-

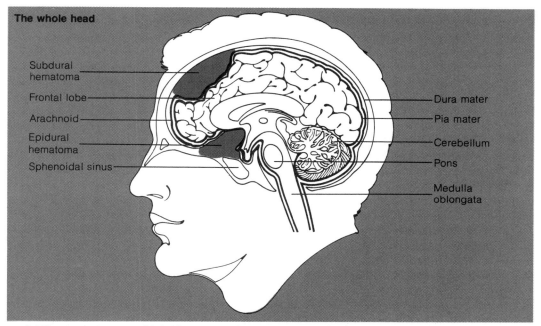

The whole head

Subdural hematoma

Frontal lobe

Arachnoid

Epidural hematoma

Sphenoidal sinus

Dura mater

Pia mater

Cerebellum

Pons

Medulla oblongata

ated. These two types of injuries cause the most severe brain damage.

What about Randy's case?

Randy obviously suffered a coup-contrecoup type injury when he was thrown from his motorcycle. But you can't tell how severely his brain was damaged until the doctor examines skull X-rays, the results of an arteriogram, computerized axial tomography (CAT), and possibly other tests.

Randy may have some type of intracranial hemorrhage or a tentorial herniation. This can lead to increasing intracranial pressure — which is always dangerous — and sometimes requires immediate surgery.

To help you review the differences between the complications and the symptoms they cause, I've listed several types below:

• *Subdural hematoma.* An accumulation of blood from a torn bridging-vein on the brain's surface; most commonly found over the frontal and temporal lobes where it may affect motor and language centers. Since the clot can form slowly, symptoms suggesting hematoma may not appear for days or

Focus on fractures
The X-rays on the opposite page show some of the skull fractures you may see in the E.D. A linear fracture (Figure 1) is a break in the bone so simple that it does not alter the relationship of the parts of the skull. A comminuted fracture (Figure 2) involves several linear fractures that interrupt the skull.

The smaller circle in Figure 2 shows a depressed fragment. Depressed fractures (Figures 3 and 4) involve the displacement of comminuted fragments.

even weeks after the head injury. Sometimes the patient and his family won't even remember the accident, because it seemed so slight. An acute subdural hematoma — which requires immediate attention — usually occurs from heavy venous bleeding after a severe head injury. To remove any hematoma, the doctor usually aspirates it through a burr hole, or with intracranial surgery.

• *Epidural hematoma.* A rapid but rare accumulation of blood between the skull and dura mater, usually caused by damage to the middle meningeal artery. Since blood loss is severe, the patient needs immediate surgical aspiration of the hematoma to save his life.

• *Tentorial herniation.* Consider this complication to be an even greater emergency than epidural hematoma. Herniation occurs when injured brain tissue swells and forces itself through the tentorial notch. This squeezes the brain stem (which passes through the notch), compresses vital centers, and cuts off the brain's blood supply. As an emergency measure, the patient is given mannitol and steroids I.V. to reduce cerebral edema and shrink brain tissue. He'll also need surgery. Symptoms vary depending on the injury's location. Look for drowsiness, confusion, dilation of one or both pupils, Cheyne-Stokes respirations, nuchal rigidity and bradycardia. Symptoms grow progressively worse with such swiftness that you may not even be aware of herniation before the patient has suffered irreversible brain damage.

Obviously, you must be aware of these complications and be able to recognize them in a head-injured patient. That takes close observation — while you're giving him the immediate care he needs — as well as an adequate neurological assessment. The doctor depends on your skill in this area to help him make his diagnosis. Watch your patient closely and be alert for any changes.

Now let's get back to Randy, so I can list the priorities you must follow with a head-injured patient. The first, of course, is to establish an adequate airway and maintain a close watch on the rate and quality of his respirations. Randy is breathing adequately, as I said earlier. *But if his breathing changed in any way, you would notify the doctor immediately.* Adequate respiration depends on a properly functioning respiratory center in the brain, and increasing intracranial pressure can cause rapid deterioration. *Nursing tip:* To clear a head-injured

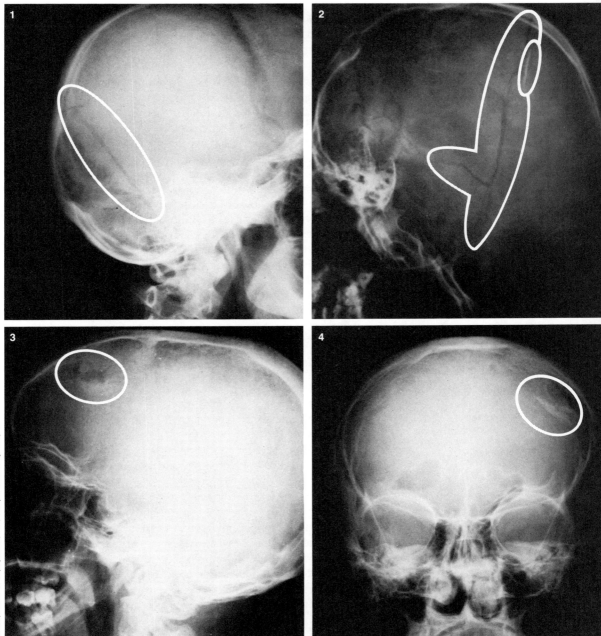

Neurologic checklist

LEVEL OF CONSCIOUSNESS
1. Alert and wakeful
2. Lethargy or restlessness
3. Orientation
    a. time
    b. place
    c. person
    d. self
4. Response to simple commands
5. Response to painful stimuli
    a. purposeful
    b. nonpurposeful
    c. no response
6. Reflexes
    a. corneal reflex
    b. gag reflex

ABILITY TO MOVE
1. Arms and legs
2. Facial muscles
3. Unusual movements
4. Babinski sign

PUPIL RESPONSES
1. Appearance
    a. shape
    b. size
    c. equality
2. Reaction to light
    a. direct reflex
    b. consensual reflex
3. Unusual eye movements

VITAL SIGNS
1. Respiration
2. Blood pressure
3. Pulse
4. Temperature

patient's airway, aspirate through his mouth. Nasal aspiration may induce leakage of spinal fluid through the nearby cribriform plate.

What next? As soon as you rule out or stabilize a cervical injury, put the patient in the correct position. To perform a quick assessment or deliver cardiopulmonary resuscitation, you may want to place a head-injured patient on his back; otherwise, put him far over on either side or on his abdomen in a swimmer's position. This prevents his tongue from occluding his airway and allows natural drainage of secretions. Remember, if you notice spinal fluid leaking from his nose or ears, keep his head raised 30°. *Caution:* Whenever you care for a patient with a head injury, never place his head lower than the rest of his body. In a case of hypovolemic shock, let his head stay elevated and raise his limbs as much as possible to increase venous return to the heart.

How do you treat spinal fluid leaks? Randy, as you recall, seems to have this complication with his injury. So you already have his head elevated 30° to put his brain at atmospheric pressure and promote spontaneous healing.

How can you be sure the leak is spinal fluid? Test it with Clinistix. Spinal fluid tests positive for sugar, mucus does not. Another way to test for spinal fluid is the "halo" sign. On bed linen, spinal fluid usually shows up as a slightly blood-tinged center spot surrounded by a lighter-colored ring. Anytime you're in doubt, put aside stained linen so the doctor can examine it.

To further care for a patient with a spinal leak, follow these guidelines:

• Keep the patient on absolute bedrest in the correct position. Instruct him not to change his position in any way.

• Is his nose running? Show him how to wipe it with a 4″ x 4″ gauze pad. Instruct him not to blow it or pick at it.

• Is his ear draining? Cover it lightly with a sterile gauze pad, changing it periodically to examine it for drainage. Do not put any packing inside the ear.

Completing the neurologic checklist

Once these priorities are taken care of, you can begin to assess the patient using the neurologic checklist. You'll find this in a simple-to-follow outline form on this page. You may want to copy it for handy reference later. But for now, let's take the steps one at a time, so I can review them with you in greater detail.

Level of consciousness. Is the patient alert and wakeful? A fully conscious person is well-oriented to his environment and responds appropriately to requests and events. Lethargy, restlessness, and irritability may be early symptoms of increasing intracranial pressure. But ask the patient's family how he normally acts: Then you'll have a baseline for comparison.

Is the patient oriented? When a person becomes disoriented he loses correct sense of himself, the place he's in, and the time. If he's conscious, start by asking him his name. Then ask him where he is. He may not know the name of the institution right away, but does he know he's in a hospital? For a further test, see if he knows the approximate date, the year, the season, or any particular holiday that may have just gone by or is about to arrive. *Nursing tip:* Remember, these questions may seem silly to the patient who *is* oriented. Explain why you must ask them — to determine the severity of his injury.

Does the patient respond to simple commands? Ask him to do such things as squeeze your hand, raise his arm, wiggle his toes, open his mouth, or touch his ear. Try him with several different commands — one at a time — to involve both sides of his body. Remember, impaired motor function, rather than lowered consciousness, may account for his inability to respond. You'll use these commands later on when you check his ability to move.

Does he respond to pain? In an unconscious patient, apply supraorbital pressure, press your fingernails into his nailbed, or firmly pinch the trapezius muscle-ridge between his neck and shoulder. Normally, the patient will respond purposefully, by trying to withdraw from the stimulus or push it away from him. At a lower level of consciousness, he'll respond nonpurposefully. For example, he may only grimace or move his body in an irrelevant fashion. A patient who is paralyzed or comatose will have no response.

Does he have corneal or gag reflexes? Reflexes are among the last responses to go. For the patient's safety, check his corneal and gag reflexes in this manner: For the corneal reflex, hold each eyelid open and lightly stroke the cornea with the tip of a gauze pad. If he doesn't blink immediately, he'll need eye care to prevent drying and irritation. For the gag reflex, hold down his tongue with a wooden depressor and touch the back of his pharynx on each side with a cotton swab. If the patient doesn't gag, provide suctioning, as needed, and watch him closely to prevent airway obstruction.

Ability to move. Injury to the patient's head or spinal cord will affect his ability to move. If you haven't already seen him move his limbs spontaneously, ask him to do so using the simple commands I mentioned earlier. To see if he has weakness or paralysis on one side, ask him to squeeze your hands. Then try to determine if each handgrip is equal in strength.

Check the movement of facial muscles. Ask the patient to smile, show you his teeth, shut his eyes tightly, or wrinkle his forehead. Watch closely for any asymmetry: for example, drooping of one eyelid, drooling, or drooping of one corner of his mouth.

Record any unusual movements and clearly describe them. This includes reflex sucking, grasping, spontaneous rigidity, rigidity in response to pain, yawning, hiccoughing, and convulsive activity.

Test to see if the Babinski sign is present, which after 18 months of age is considered abnormal and indicates brain damage.

Pupil responses. Check the patient's pupils for equality of size, reaction to light, and consensual reflex. Keep in mind, though, that many healthy people have slightly unequal pupils. Remember too that a direct blow to the eye, as well as some medications, will impair pupillary responses.

Record and describe any unusual eye movements: for example, deviation of one or both eyes from midline, back-and-forth oscillation, or bilateral deviation toward the center.

Stay alert for seizures

As you assess your head-injured patient, be prepared in case he has a seizure. Don't panic. Stay with him and ask someone to call the doctor for you.

Don't waste time searching for a padded tongue depressor for his mouth. Turn the patient on his side, protect him from injury, and maintain a patent airway, if possible. Observe the seizure closely, then record its duration, when it started, which limbs moved, any incontinence, or any unusual posturing. Watch and record the patient's reactions *after* the seizure. The doctor will want a detailed description of all you've observed.

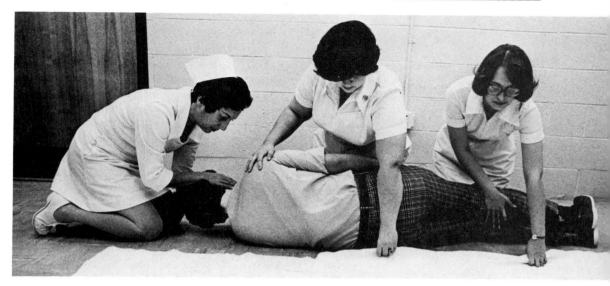

Spinal injuries

So far, I've discussed head injuries. As you know, an accident victim may also have suffered serious spinal injury. In fact, each year such injuries cause total paralysis in more than 10,000 people in the U.S. and Canada.

Fractures and dislocations of the spine are dangerous because they can damage the spinal cord and meninges. Crushing, cutting, or severing of the cord can happen at any point along the vertebral column, but the risk is greater if the fracture occurs in one of the cervical vertebrae. In that area, the spinal cord is relatively large—and thus more vulnerable.

Severity of damage depends on the type of injury and the kind of care the patient receives immediately after the accident. For example, if a patient's cord is severed at the fifth cervical vertebra, his body below that point will probably be permanently paralyzed. If the patient's cord is crushed, his neurologic deficits may not be that devastating. Below the level of injury, he'll suffer impaired motor and sensory function, but his condition may be reversible.

Any time you suspect a patient has spinal injury, call the doctor at once, then follow these priorities:

• Immobilize him immediately, using whatever equipment you have—for example, sandbags, an immobilization board, or a hard cervical collar—and see that X-rays are taken. If the

Roll like a log

If you must move a patient with a suspected spinal injury, avoid flexing his back, as in the photograph above, since this may further injure the spinal column.

To turn a patient in bed, place his arms across his chest. Tell him to hold himself rigid except for his legs. Place a pillow between his knees to reduce pressure.

When you move the patient to the side of the bed, keep his spinal column rigid by holding the turn sheet as taut as possible. This will enable you to turn the patient as though you were rolling a log. Once the patient has turned, you may allow him to flex his upper leg supported by a pillow, to make him more comfortable.

patient is brought to the E.D. on a board, let him remain on it while the X-rays are being taken. Never try to move a patient with a spinal injury unless you know how to do it properly and have enough people to help you (see page 127).

• Establish an open airway and pay close attention to the patient's breathing. If his respirations become rapid and shallow with flaring of the nostrils, suspect trouble. Get help immediately.

• Assess the patient's condition by getting his history and asking him exactly how the accident happened. If the patient is unconscious or unable to answer questions, get the information from his family or whoever accompanied him. Evaluate the extent of his injuries by completing the neurologic checklist on page 124.

• Control any external hemorrhage from concurrent injuries.

• Watch closely for symptoms of spinal shock, which occurs when the muscles below the injury level are completely paralyzed. Autonomic nervous system activity is blocked, causing blood pressure to drop rapidly. Reflexes that control bladder and gastrointestinal system functions are gone, and the patient suffers urinary retention and gastric distention. An abrupt onset of fever occurs because the patient no longer perspires on the paralyzed portion of his body.

When spinal shock seems inevitable, do the following: Start an I.V. with the appropriate solution; insert a Foley catheter to prevent urinary retention; and see that the patient has a nasogastric tube to reduce gastric distention.

• Comfort and reassure the patient as much as possible, so he won't become panicky. Explain why he's been immobilized; assure him that you are doing everything you can to help him. Never use morphine to sedate a patient with a spinal injury. Morphine, as you know, depresses respirations.

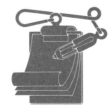

Remember these important points when caring for a patient with a head or spinal injury:
1. Consider a brain contusion more serious than a concussion.
2. When caring for a spine-injured patient, be alert for signs and symptoms of spinal shock.
3. To differentiate leaking spinal fluid from other secretions, look for the halo sign on bed linens, or test the secretion with a Clinistix.
4. Be sure to record and describe any unusual movements.

SKILLCHECK
5

1. Sixty-year-old Bertha Estus is brought to the emergency department of the hospital, where you work, with a severe nosebleed. She says it came on suddenly from no apparent cause. Her daughter, Faye, who has accompanied her, tells you that her mother has frequent nosebleeds. "They seem to be getting a lot worse," she says. "I think my mother should see a doctor." What do you do first?

2. Kenneth Markel, a 42-year-old doorman, has spent the past two days in bed with a sore throat. When he finally keeps an appointment with the doctor, he complains that his throat pain seems much worse. His voice is extremely raspy and you can see that he's having great difficulty swallowing. You take his temperature and find that it's 104° F. (40° C.). What does this suggest to you and what do you do about it?

3. Gardening is Anna Malone's favorite hobby. Her hybrid rose garden attracts many visitors to her yard and gives Mrs. Malone great pleasure. However, one day, a large Japanese beetle flies into her ear and becomes lodged there — causing Mrs. Malone severe pain. Her neighbor brings her to the clinic, where you work, for immediate treatment. Mrs. Malone is screaming when you see her and clutching her ear. How can you help her?

4. You're doing a neurological assessment on 34-year-old Donald Hemple, who was rushed to the emergency department after suffering severe head injuries in a fall from his horse. You've just completed checking his level of consciousness, his ability to move, and his response to pain. You're about to examine his pupil responses, when suddenly Mr. Hemple has a seizure. What do you do now?

5. Buck DeWitt has won numerous trophies in competitive swim meets. He practices daily in the school pool and gives swimming lessons at a local country club. However, one day Buck suffers serious injuries in a diving accident. Because the ambulance attendants that arrive on the scene suspect Buck has a spinal injury, they place him on an immobilization board before rushing him to the hospital. What do you do first to help Buck when he arrives in the emergency department?

6. Halfway through a performance of Guys and Dolls, 20-year-old Lenny Segal falls 15 feet from the stage into the orchestra pit. He's immediately rushed to the emergency department of the hospital where you are a triage nurse. When you see Lenny, he's unconscious, but breathing adequately. However, you notice a small amount of clear fluid leaking from his nose and right ear. What do you do next?

7. Leslie Davenport, a 16-year-old high school student, accepts a ride home from a girlfriend who has just learned to drive. Despite numerous warnings from Leslie, her friend loses control of the car on an icy country road and smashes into a tree. The girlfriend is killed instantly and Leslie is thrown forward, hitting the dashboard. When you see Leslie in the emergency department of the hospital not long after that, she's suffering severe face and neck pain and whispers that it's difficult to swallow. You note that the skin covering her larynx feels swollen and seems like it's stretched over crumpled cellophane. What emergency care do you give to her?

(Answers on page 184)

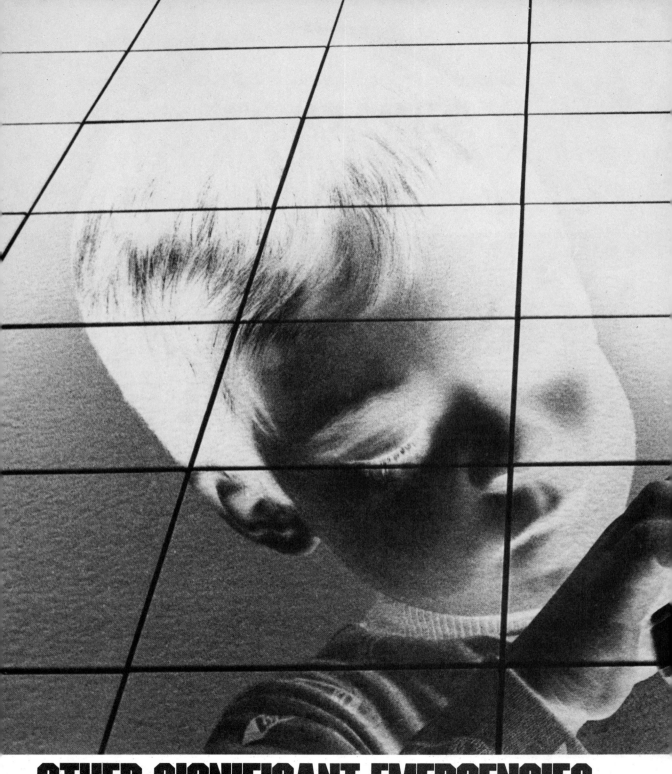

OTHER SIGNIFICANT EMERGENCIES

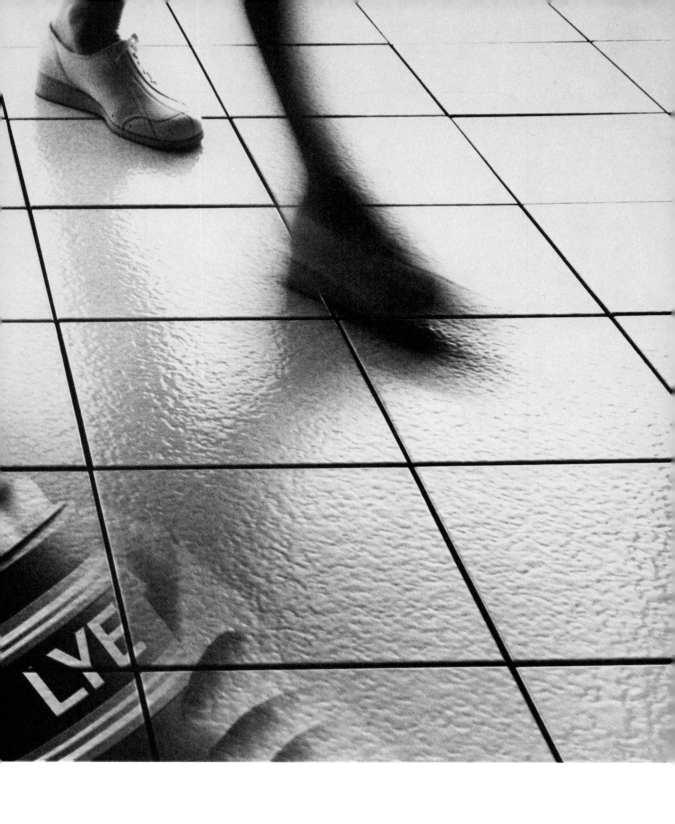

What nursing actions should you take when a patient's signs and symptoms suggest the possibility of hypovolemic shock?

If your patient's depressed after a mastectomy, what can you do to help?

What emergency actions do you take when a patient swallows a petroleum product or corrosive acid?

If a patient with severe burns passes black urine, what should you suspect?

What can you do to increase absorption of epinephrine in a patient with anaphylactic shock?

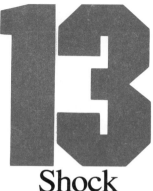

Shock

How to defeat the tricky killer

MINNIE ROSE, RN, BSN, MEd

"HE WAS CUTTING BACK our lilac bush when he slipped on some wet grass and fell on the electric hedge clipper," Mrs. Baker cries. You've just met her at the door of the emergency department, where she and a neighbor have rushed her 33-year-old husband, Michael.

You realize his right thigh must be deeply lacerated because the towels they've wrapped around his leg are saturated with blood. With the help of the neighbor and another nurse, you get Mr. Baker on a stretcher and call for a doctor.

Working quickly as a team, you take Mr. Baker's vital signs while the other nurse applies pressure to the hemorrhaging area with sterile pads. His blood pressure is 88/50, his pulse 132, and his respirations 34. His skin feels cold and clammy, and he seems very weak.

What do you do next? Mr. Baker's already showing signs of hypovolemic — or hemorrhagic — shock. And he'll require vigorous treatment to keep his condition from becoming irreversible. Do you know what priorities to follow when a patient develops hypovolemic shock? What do you do for patients with other forms of shock: septic, cardiogenic, neurogenic? Are you skilled enough to stay ahead of any shock condition that's likely to occur? If you're even slightly uncertain, you need the information in this chapter.

What causes shock?
One major deficit is peculiar to all forms of shock. That deficit is inadequate tissue perfusion caused by failure of the circulatory system to function as it should. Circulation, as you know, depends on the proper balance of the following: volume of circulating blood, vascular resistance, and effective cardiac output.

A temporary shift in the balance of these three components occurs as different physical needs arise. For example, the heart can beat faster and harder to meet increased oxygen needs during exercise.

But suppose a profound shift in balance occurs — as it would if a patient had a massive hemorrhage? Unless this shift was compensated for in some way, the patient's circulatory system would cease to function properly, and inadequate tissue perfusion would result.

Blood volume loss isn't the only thing that can upset circulatory balance, however. As I said above, circulation also depends on the following: vascular resistance and adequate cardiac output. So a weak or inefficient heartbeat could trigger circulatory malfunction, and so could sudden dilation of the blood vessels. The triggering mechanism is what classifies the shock by type, as you can see in the chart on page 135.

Staying ahead of a killer
Look for shock in any condition where it's a likely complication: for example, severe injuries of all types, loss of blood or body fluids, infection, or heart failure.

By anticipating shock before it occurs, you'll be ready to treat it. And that will give you an advantage in your fight against a killer. Shock is tricky to treat because the treatment must always be double-barreled. You must control the condition that caused the shock, as well as the shock itself.

Watch for these signs and symptoms
Remember, no patient's shock ever develops exactly like the classic textbook examples. But you can still rely on the appearance of certain symptoms — with few exceptions — in every major type of shock. Look for:

MAJOR TYPES OF SHOCK		
TRIGGERING MECHANISM	WHERE IT OCCURS	THIS TYPE OF SHOCK RESULTS
Abnormal loss of fluid caused by hemorrhage, severe burns, diarrhea, etc.	Bloodstream or tissue cells	Hypovolemic
Weak, inefficient beat or heart failure caused by myocardial infarction, cardiac tamponade, etc.	Heart	Cardiogenic
Cell destruction from endotoxins caused by bacterial infection (usually gram-negative)	Tissue	Septic
Abnormal dilation of blood vessels caused by cervical fracture, concussion, spinal cord injury, or spinal anesthesia	Blood vessels	Neurogenic

• decreased temperature, except in early septic shock. (In early septic shock, the patient's temperature is elevated. In late septic shock, however, his temperature drops to subnormal.)

• tachycardia with weak, thready pulse

• rapid, shallow respirations. Air hunger forces the body to try to compensate for tissue anoxia. In most types of shock, slow breathing appears *late* — after failure of this compensatory mechanism. In septic shock, the patient's respiration rate increases *markedly* as his condition worsens.

• hypotension with a narrowing of pulse pressure. Systolic pressure falls before diastolic, producing the narrowed pulse pressure.

• skin changes: changes in skin temperature and color reflect tissue oxygenation and perfusion. Skin may feel cold and clammy, except in early septic shock when it may feel warm and flushed. Pallor and cyanosis may indicate tissue hypoxia, though cyanosis in lips and nail beds also occurs if a patient is cold. To avoid confusion, check for cyanosis in an extremity that's lightly covered. Since *change* is the key, the same nurse should check the patient for cyanosis each time.

Some drugs commonly used in shock

ADRENERGICS
dobutamine hydrochloride (Dobutrex): 250-mg vial diluted and added to 250, 500, or 1,000 ml of dextrose 5% in water. Titrate drip rate to 2.5 to 10 mcg/kg/minute.

dopamine hydrochloride (Intropin): 200- or 400-mg ampul added to 250 or 500 ml dextrose 5% in water, normal saline solution, combination of dextrose and saline solution, or lactated Ringer's injection. Titrate to 2 to 5 mcg/kg/minute up to 50 mcg/kg/minute.

norepinephrine injection (Levophed): Initially 8 to 12 mcg/-minute by I.V. infusion. Average maintenance dose 2 to 4 mcg/minute.

metaraminol bitartrate (Aramine): 0.5 to 5 mg I.V. bolus followed by 15 to 100 mg in 500 ml of normal saline or dextrose 5% in water. Titrate infusion rate to desired blood pressure reading.

In a dark-skinned patient, check for cyanosis by pressing lightly on his fingernail, earlobe, or lips. In cyanosis, tissue color won't return within the normal, 1-second interval. Color will return from the periphery only. Normally, it returns from below the pale spot, as well.

Caution: Never rely on good skin color as proof of adequate tissue oxygenation. Have an arterial blood sample drawn to measure the oxygen level.

• diminished urinary output because of decreased circulation to kidneys
• restlessness, confusion, and anxiety, caused by inadequate oxygenation of brain. As shock deepens, the patient may become apathetic, delirious, or comatose.
• increased thirst.

Setting your goals

As I indicated earlier, shock can be very difficult to treat, because you must control the condition that caused the shock, as well as the shock itself. To do both successfully, individualize the patient's care and reevaluate his condition several times an hour. Be sure to document your observations completely.

Treatment, of course, varies with each type of shock. But keep in mind that the three shock care priorities remain constant: adequate ventilation, adequate circulation, and adequate urinary output (at least 30 ml/hour).

In the next few pages, I'll discuss the differences between the major types of shock. (Anaphylactic shock is reviewed at length in Chapter 16.)

Michael Baker: A patient in hypovolemic shock

As you recall from the beginning of this chapter, Michael Baker was rushed to the hospital hemorrhaging from a deep laceration on his thigh. His blood pressure had dropped to 88/50, his pulse was 132 and thready, and his respiratory rate was 34. You've already felt his skin, and it was cold and clammy. You now note that he's still conscious, but he seems very weak.

What do you do next? Put Mr. Baker flat on his back. He's already displaying the classic signs of hypovolemic shock, which in his case was triggered by his massive hemorrhage.

Hemorrhage, of course, is one of the leading causes of

hypovolemic shock — though the hemorrhage may not always be as obvious as Mr. Baker's. As you know, severe blood loss can occur internally; for example, from gastrointestinal disease or from traumatic injury. Massive fluid loss, another cause of hypovolemic shock, can occur from peritonitis, severe burns, or diarrhea.

Normally, a patient's body can compensate for a 10% loss of blood or fluid by constricting arteriolar beds, increasing heart rate and force of contractions, and redistributing fluids. During this period, the patient's vital signs, skin color, and skin temperature will probably remain normal. (His cardiac output, of course, will be slightly reduced.)

However, by the time blood or fluid loss reaches 15% to 25%, the picture changes. The patient can no longer compensate for the circulatory insult, and he begins to show symptoms of hypovolemic shock.

What happens is this. Generalized vasoconstriction sharply reduces the blood flow to the vital organs (brain, kidneys, liver, and lungs), as well as to peripheral muscle. As a result, cells no longer receive the oxygen they need and form increased quantities of lactic acid.

Because renal and hepatic functions have been impaired by vasoconstriction, this lactic acid can't be broken down and removed from the bloodstream. The accumulated acidic waste eventually overwhelms the patient's internal buffer system, and metabolic acidosis results.

To compensate for metabolic acidosis, the patient hyperventilates to bring more oxygen to the tissues, and in doing so creates respiratory alkalosis. But no matter how strong he is, he can maintain the physical exertion of hyperventilation for only a short time. Eventually he needs some respiratory support — either oxygen by mask or mechanical ventilation. (Shock patients who don't hyperventilate during this period have a higher chance of respiratory failure.)

To stay ahead of shock, then, you can't just watch for signs of cyanosis. These may not occur till later on, when shock is no longer easily reversible. Instead, start administering a low percentage of oxygen immediately when the patient's condition suggests the possibility of hypovolemic shock. The doctor will probably want a blood sample drawn, to measure the patient's blood-gas levels at regular intervals. (For a list of normal blood-gas levels, see page 62.)

Some drugs commonly used in shock

DIGITALIS GLYCOSIDES
digoxin (Lanoxin): 0.5 to 1 mg I.V.

deslanoside (Cedilanid-D): 1.2 to 1.6 mg I.V. in divided doses over 24 hours

SYSTEMIC BUFFER
sodium bicarbonate: 7.5% or 8.4% solution, 1 to 3 mEq/kg I.V.

ANTIHISTAMINE
diphenhydramine (Benadryl): 50 to 100 mg I.V., 50 mg P.O. every 6 hours

SPASMOLYTIC AGENT
aminophylline: 500 mg in 250 ml dextrose 5% in water (2 mg/2.2 kg of body weight)

CORTICOSTEROIDS
dexamethasone phosphate (Decadron Phosphate): 1 to 6 mg/kg I.V. single dose or 40 mg I.V. every 2 to 6 hours, as necessary

hydrocortisone (Solu-Cortef): 500 mg to 2 g every 2 to 6 hours

Since massive blood or fluid loss can occur internally as well as externally, always assume a trauma victim is in hypovolemic shock, until you can prove otherwise. In some situations, the doctor may apply antishock trousers (for more details, see page 52). Be prepared to perform the following emergency care priorities, as ordered by the doctor:

• Place the patient flat on his back to ease circulatory resistance.

• Check for an open airway and adequate circulation and start cardiopulmonary resuscitation, if necessary.

• Administer low-percentage (24%) oxygen by face mask or airway to ensure adequate oxygenation of tissues. Later, you can adjust the oxygen flow to a higher level if blood-gas measurements indicate the need.

• At the same time, start I.V.s in both arms or legs with lactated Ringer's solution or normal saline, using a large-bore catheter. The large-bore catheter will make it easier for you to administer any needed blood transfusions later.

Caution: When you start I.V.s in a shock patient who's suffered abdominal trauma, don't use his legs for infusion sites. If you do, the fluid may escape through the ruptured vessels into his abdomen.

How much fluid to give can't be determined at first, of course. The doctor will have to insert a central venous pressure (CVP) line or Swan-Ganz catheter to monitor circulating blood volume.

• Insert a Foley catheter to measure urine output, another good indicator of adequate fluid balance. Output should be greater than 50 ml/hour in adults. If it isn't, increase the fluid infusion rate but watch for signs of overhydration. Notify the doctor if the patient's urine output still does not improve.

• Have an arterial blood sample drawn to measure blood-gas levels and have venous blood drawn for a complete blood count (CBC), electrolytes, type, and crossmatch.

• Keep the patient covered with a light blanket. Do not overheat, which may increase his metabolic rate and need for oxygen.

• Record his blood pressure, pulse rate, and other vital signs every 15 minutes. A systolic blood pressure below 80 mm Hg usually indicates inadequate coronary artery blood flow, which may produce weak contractions and cardiac arrhythmias. When his blood pressure drops this low, increase the oxygen rate and call the doctor immediately. A progressive drop in blood pressure accompanied by a thready pulse usually indicates inadequate fluid replacement. Notify the doctor and increase the infusion rate.

• Observe the patient's skin color and temperature and note any changes. Cold, clammy skin during fluid replacement is a sign of continuing peripheral vascular constriction. The doctor will probably want you to increase the infusion rate.

In many cases, you'll be able to reverse hypovolemic shock with prompt, adequate fluid replacement, oxygen, and careful monitoring of vital signs. Although vasoconstrictors increase blood pressure, they aren't always the treatment of choice (see page 50).

Cardiogenic shock: Another look at Mr. Frankenfeld
Cardiogenic shock is caused by the heart's failure to pump properly. It's the leading cause of death among patients hospitalized for acute myocardial infarction. Cardiogenic shock occurs in about 15% of these patients, and the mortality rate is estimated at about 85%. It can also develop secondary to cardiac tamponade or pulmonary embolus.

You remember Mr. Frankenfeld from Chapter 4, don't you? Well, he could have gone into cardiogenic shock at any time after he suffered his MI. With cardiogenic shock, a patient displays the same generalized signs as a patient with any other type of shock. But these signs may also suggest congestive heart failure, making an accurate assessment of his condition very difficult.

You'd have suspected cardiogenic shock if Mr. Frankenfeld developed any of the following: decreased urinary output, blood pressure changes, narrowing of pulse pressure, pulmonary rales, or a gallop heart rhythm. He may also have been extremely pale with cool, clammy skin. These symptoms may have appeared gradually, but you noticed them because you were monitoring the patient closely.

If cardiogenic shock develops in a patient, the doctor will probably order dopamine (Intropin). This acts as a vasoconstrictor on the skeletal-muscle blood vessels, but dilates cardiac, renal, and mesenteric vessels. This has a positive inotropic effect on the myocardium, causing an increase in cardiac output, renal blood flow, glomerular filtration, and urine production. However, these effects are dose-related; high doses cause opposite effects.

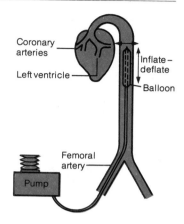

A pump of life
A device used increasingly in the care of cardiogenic shock is the intra-aortic balloon pump. You should familiarize yourself with how it functions and what nursing care it involves so you can explain the procedure to your patient.

During surgery the doctor inserts the balloon pump through the femoral artery into the patient's descending thoracic aorta. He sets it to follow the action of the patient's heart. By inflating during diastole, the pump increases perfusion of vital organs and oxygenation of the myocardium. By deflating immediately before systole, it reduces the workload and metabolic needs of the heart.

After the catheter is inserted, watch for signs of arterial occlusion or an interrupted blood supply to the involved leg. Check popliteal, tibial, and dorsalis pedis pulses every 15 minutes. If you notice any irregularities, notify the doctor immediately.

**Toxic shock syndrome (TSS):
Not for women only**
You've probably heard this condition referred to as the tampon-
user's disease. However, as
we've learned more about this
elusive syndrome, we've found it
affects men and children, too.

Caused by a toxin produced
by *Staphylococcus aureus,* the
signs and symptoms include
high fever (above 102° F.,
38.9° C.), diarrhea, vomiting, and
erythroderma (sunburn-type
rash), which later desquamates.
Eventually, the patient experi-
ences confusion, syncope, and
shock. He may also exhibit signs
of acute renal failure, cardiac
enlargement, mild disseminated
intravascular coagulation (DIC),
or acute respiratory distress
syndrome (ARDS). Laboratory
tests also may confirm pyuria,
hypocalcemia, and thrombocyto-
penia.

Because TTS resembles septic
shock, many of your previous
patients with this condition were
actually diagnosed as septic
shock victims. The differentiating
factor, however, is the TSS patient does not have bacteremia
or a disseminated infection. Also,
diarrhea and the diffuse sunburn-
type rash are rarely exhibited
by the patient in septic shock.

What can you do? Be alert for
the signs and symptoms; you
may be the first one to recognize
the condition. You'll also play a
major role in therapy, by administering (on doctor's orders) large
volumes of normal saline solution
or lactated Ringer's solution,
penicillinase-resistant penicillins,
and high doses of corticosteroids. Careful monitoring of blood
pressure with an arterial line
and frequent urinary output determination are other supportive
measures you'll perform. Also
be alert for the onset of these
complications: acute renal failure, ARDS, DIC, and hepatic
failure.

Caution: Dopamine can cause sloughing and necrosis near
the injection site by infiltration of surrounding tissue. To prevent this, start the I.V. in a large vein — preferably one in the
antecubital fossa — not a vein in the hand, wrist or ankle. If
drug infiltration occurs, stop the infusion immediately and call
the doctor.

Depending on his response to dopamine, a patient may need
his dosage adjusted. If his blood pressure elevates excessively, his dosage may have to be reduced or discontinued.

Whenever a doctor orders a vasopressor like dopamine,
watch for wide swings in blood pressure and check for fluid
overload. Stop the drug immediately if the patient develops
signs of toxicity: headache, chest pain, or premature ventricular contractions.

Continue to watch the patient carefully, and report any
changes in his condition to the doctor. If you're administering
fluids, be alert for signs of fluid overload: dyspnea, cough,
rhonchi, or rales. Don't rely on central venous pressure (CVP)
monitoring to tell if the patient has fluid overload, because it
doesn't accurately measure left-ventricular pressure. Instead,
measure pulmonary artery pressure (PAP) or pulmonary
wedge pressure (PWP) with a Swan-Ganz catheter.

Septic shock: Can you beat the high mortality rate?
Perhaps the major difference between the course of
hypovolemic shock and that of septic shock is time. In
hypovolemic shock, the progression from hypotension to ischemia to anoxia usually takes several hours — time enough to
stop bleeding and start fluid replacement in most patients.

However, in septic shock, anoxia can develop in less than
an hour — sometimes even seconds. How fast depends on two
things: the amount of endotoxin released by bacteria (usually
gram-negative) that have invaded the bloodstream, and the
patient's susceptibility.

Certain patients run a greater risk than others of developing
septic shock: newborns, patients over age 60, all debilitated
patients, diabetics, cancer patients who've undergone
chemotherapy or whole-body radiation, patients with open
wounds or abscesses, surgery patients, patients on im-
munosuppressive medication, and catheterized patients.

Pay close attention to patients in these high-risk categories.
And remember that septic shock develops somewhat differ-

ently from other forms of shock. In the early stages, the patient's skin may feel warm and dry, instead of cold and clammy. His urine output may be normal or even excessive, instead of diminished.

Call the doctor at once if the patient develops *any* of these signs or symptoms:

• low-grade fever (100° F. to 101° F.), except in burn patients, who may be hypothermic

• blunted sensorium (inability to concentrate, increasing confusion)

• increased pulse rate and respirations

• hypotension (may be slight at first, but will become marked as shock progresses)

• diminished urine output

• warm, dry skin. As shock progresses, the skin becomes cold and clammy

• gastrointestinal symptoms (nausea, vomiting, cramps, or distention)

• elevated white blood cell count (WBC), increased blood urea nitrogen (BUN), and proteinuria. Blood-gas measurements show a trend toward metabolic acidosis, unless the patient is hyperventilating, in which case the measurements will show alkalosis.

Begin treatment immediately, remembering that it must be directed at the cause of the infection, as well as the shock itself. To do this, the doctor will probably order the following:

• A broad-spectrum antibiotic, such as carbenicillin or gentamicin to fight infection, until the cause can be determined by culture. *Nursing tip:* If you give the patient both carbenicillin and gentamicin, take care not to give them at the same time. Carbenicillin may inactivate gentamicin. Always space them 2 to 4 hours apart.

• A steroid, such as dexamethasone or hydrocortisone, to reduce inflammation and to improve cardiovascular function. When endotoxin is released in the bloodstream, it causes intense vasospasm in the small vessels, particularly those in the liver, kidneys, and lungs.

• I.V. fluid replacement, with titration based on the patient's urinary output, blood pressure, pulse rate, and central venous pressure.

• Oxygen, as needed, to support respiration.

As you know, the mortality rate for septic shock remains

high (about 80%). But it doesn't have to be, if you stay alert for signs and symptoms in high-risk patients.

Neurogenic shock

Compared with other forms of shock, neurogenic shock is rare. In the emergency department, you'll see it only in patients with concussions, cervical fractures, or spinal cord injuries. Elsewhere in the hospital, it can occur from spinal anesthesia, which blocks the sympathetic nervous system.

What triggers neurogenic shock? Injury or anesthesia abnormally dilates the patient's peripheral vessels, decreasing his blood pressure and permitting blood to pool in his venous beds.

Despite this hypotension, the patient usually shows signs of good tissue perfusion and may stay alert—unless his head injury has altered his level of consciousness.

What can you do for a patient who develops neurogenic shock? Keep him flat (*never* in Trendelenburg position), and continue to administer fluids, as described in Chapter 12.

Since extreme pain can precipitate neurogenic shock in patients with severe head or spinal injuries, the doctor may also order a drug to relieve pain without depressing respirations.

Remember these important points when caring for a patient in shock:

1. Be alert for signs and symptoms of hypovolemic shock in a patient who's experienced a massive fluid loss, such as external or internal hemorrhage, burns, peritonitis, or prolonged diarrhea.

2. Administer oxygen immediately to a patient with signs and symptoms of hypovolemic shock.

3. Use a Swan-Ganz catheter to measure pulmonary artery pressure (PAP) or pulmonary artery wedge pressure (PAWP).

4. Never place a patient in shock in Trendelenburg position; instead position him flat on his back.

14

Severe Burns
How to save a life in balance

CLAUDELLA A. JONES, RN, AND IRVING FELLER, MD

THOSE FIRST CRUCIAL HOURS...they're the most important when you're caring for a severely burned patient. What you do — or fail to do — for him during the first 24 to 36 hours may tip the scales. His life will hang in the balance as you strive to keep burn shock from developing into a more dangerous condition, initiate and titrate fluid therapy, provide proper wound care, and prevent deadly infection.

How sharp are your skills for this emergency? For example, do you know which burn patients are most likely to develop serious respiratory difficulties? Do you know how to titrate fluids correctly? Do you know which patients need an electrocardiogram taken? This chapter will answer these questions and teach you how to "think emergency burn care" when you're faced with one of these critically ill patients. It'll help you supply the emotional needs of your patient during this stressful time — and cope with your own reactions to his unsightly wounds, as well.

As you probably know, treatment of the seriously burned patient falls into three phases: the emergent period (which we'll discuss in this chapter), the acute period, and the rehabilitative period. The most crucial, as we mentioned above,

is the emergent period. If you're a hospital nurse, this starts when the patient is admitted to the emergency department, where you'll:
• provide proper life-support measures.
• start fluid therapy and measure urinary output to keep burn shock from progressing to hypovolemic shock.
• clean burn wounds and treat any concurrent injuries.
• protect the patient from infection.

Setting priorities
Let's take first things first. Imagine, for example, you're a nurse in an emergency department. On a stretcher in front of you lies 19-year-old Karen McConnell, who within the last hour has been rescued from her flaming sports car. You can't yet tell the extent of her severe burns, but according to the ambulance crew, Karen was pinned in her burning car for only a minute. When you see her, she's fully conscious—though babbling somewhat incoherently about the accident. Her vital signs are stable. What do you do now?

Team effort does the job. You and another nurse must accomplish the following tasks in the next few minutes:
• Call a doctor.
• Make sure Karen has an open airway and provide humidified oxygen at a measured volume.
• With a large-bore catheter, start an I.V. to give lactated Ringer's solution and serum albumin.
• Insert a Foley catheter to measure urinary output.

We'll get into the hows and whys of the last two items a little later when we talk about fluid therapy. Right now, let's discuss respiratory support—and what problems you'll encounter with a severely burned patient like Karen.

Edema from inflammation could obstruct her breathing anytime within the first 48 hours. Expect difficulties if you see the following: face or neck burns, singed nasal hair, darkened sputum, and burn or carbon marks on the oral and nasal mucous membranes. If the patient received burns in an enclosed space—as Karen did—she probably breathed hot air, smoke or noxious chemicals. You can assume that her upper airway is damaged and most likely her lower airway, as well.

Follow this procedure if you find or anticipate respiratory problems:
• Elevate her head and torso (if blood pressure is normal).

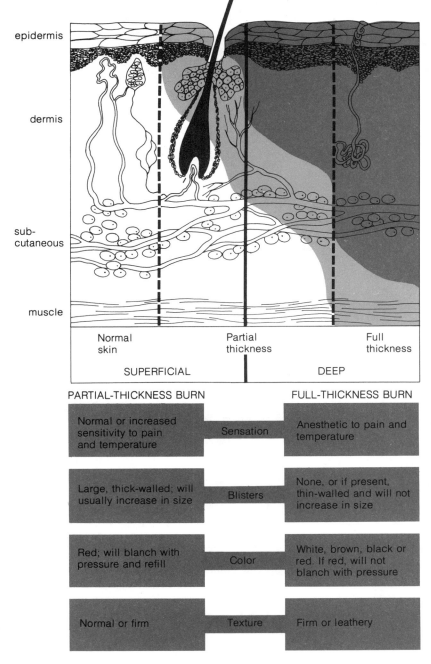

epidermis

dermis

sub-cutaneous

muscle

Normal skin	Partial thickness	Full thickness
SUPERFICIAL		DEEP

Depth of burn

In this drawing the area with dark shading shows dead tissue, while the area with light shading represents damaged tissue that will eventually heal.

Use the table below to assess the depth of burn. Then consult page 149 to determine the burn's size. These two considerations will help you determine exactly how severe the patient's burn is.

PARTIAL-THICKNESS BURN		FULL-THICKNESS BURN
Normal or increased sensitivity to pain and temperature	Sensation	Anesthetic to pain and temperature
Large, thick-walled; will usually increase in size	Blisters	None, or if present, thin-walled and will not increase in size
Red; will blanch with pressure and refill	Color	White, brown, black or red. If red, will not blanch with pressure
Normal or firm	Texture	Firm or leathery

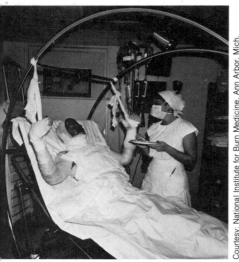

Courtesy: National Institute for Burn Medicine, Ann Arbor, Mich.

Position is everything
During the emergent period, place the patient with burns of the upper torso in a high Fowler's position. Elevate his arms with pillows, or suspend them from I.V. poles or from the frame of a CircOlectric bed. Make sure his arms are above the heart level.
This position reduces edema of the face, neck, and extremities. It also enhances the patient's circulation and decreases the heart's workload. Release the patient from this position every 2 hours for at least 30 minutes and turn him side to side.

• Ensure an open airway. Suction nasopharynx and place an endotracheal tube nearby so she can be intubated, if needed.
• Start humidified oxygen with a 40% Venti-mask.
• Tell Karen to cough and deep breathe every 2 minutes.
• Turn her from side to back to side hourly.
• Get a chest X-ray.
• Draw an arterial blood sample of 3 to 5 ml for blood-gas studies. Be sure to note on the specimen the rate and concentration of oxygen she's receiving.
• Monitor all vital signs closely and watch for signs of cerebral depression.

Remember that burns—no matter how severe—don't cause a patient to lose consciousness. If a patient like Karen is drowsy, confused, or comatose, search for other causes: sepsis, dehydration, and shock, for example.

As you'd expect, lower-airway injury (or primary pulmonary damage) is the most difficult to treat. Be ready if the doctor decides to use bronchodilators, antibiotics, or steroids to reduce the inflammatory process. Have a tracheostomy tube and tray handy even though it might not be needed. The doctor probably won't resort to a tracheostomy unless all other measures fail to relieve obstruction—or lung ventilation is impossible without it.

What else is wrong?

Now give Karen a head-to-toe check to see if anything else is wrong. Remember, she was pulled from her wrecked, burning car and she could have injuries even more critical than her burns. Keep in mind that a burn wound itself never hemorrhages. So, bleeding may mean Karen has lacerations, internal injuries, or compound fractures that require X-rays and prompt treatment.

To do a full body examination of Karen (or any patient with severe burns) remove her clothing by cutting it along the seam lines. Don't try to remove it the usual way, or you may damage burned tissue even further. If you have difficulty—or need to remove dressings that were put on at the scene—soak them in a 1:1 peroxide-saline solution or immerse Karen in a hydrotherapy tub, if her condition permits.

Let's suppose that you discover severe lacerations on Karen's right forearm. Blood oozes from the cuts onto some of the partial-thickness burns that surround them. The doctor will have to clean and suture the lacerations, but first he'll need an X-ray to make sure Karen doesn't have a fractured bone. Until that's accomplished, you should control the bleeding with a bandage. Check to be sure the bandage isn't too tight, however, to prevent further damage to the burned tissue. In addition, to prevent a paralytic ileus, insert a nasogastric tube.

Naturally, you'll check Karen's vital signs every few minutes as long as she remains in the emergency room. And you'll record information about her past medical history, allergies, and any medications she's been taking.

Now, let's consider the aggressive fluid therapy she—and all severely burned patients—will need to alleviate shock.

Fluids for burns: Why and how

Remember, the initial insult of a burn sets off the body's normal inflammatory responses. If the burn was relatively minor, the body can usually compensate for this. But if it's extensive—or present with other injuries—the body's normal homeostatic mechanisms may be compromised.

With a severe burn, the inflammatory process in the first 24 to 48 hours shifts huge amounts of fluid out of the victim's bloodstream into interstitial spaces. It does so because increased capillary permeability upsets the osmosis and diffusion that normally maintain a delicate balance. We call this shift *burn shock.* Without vigorous fluid therapy to combat it, it can easily lead to hypovolemic shock and eventual death.

Starting fluid therapy is one of the first things to do when you get a severely burned patient in the E.D. And since a doctor may not always be present immediately, you must understand how it's done. Before you start any fluids, you should know which patients should receive fluids, and what kind of fluids and how much should be given.

Who should receive fluids? Anyone with a burn larger than 20% of the total body area, anyone under age 4 or over 35, or anyone who is dehydrated, hemorrhaging, or has other injuries. Karen, as you've already discovered, needs prompt fluid therapy; she has burns over approximately 35% of her body and she also has arm lacerations.

What kind of fluids should be given? Fluid going from the bloodstream into interstitial spaces is largely plasma, so the replacement fluid should be plasma or a plasma-like substitute. Use lactated Ringer's solution because its electrolyte content approximates that of blood, and add 25 grams of serum albumin to each liter of fluid. Start the fluid in a large vein with an 18-gauge catheter. Or assist with a cutdown in any extremity.

After a few days of aggressive fluid therapy, Karen's capillary walls should return to normal. Fluids will reenter her bloodstream and start getting excreted by her kidneys. A profound diuresis occurs at this point, usually 2 to 7 days postburn, depending on the burn's severity and treatment. This diuresis signals the end of the emergent period. I.V. fluids then get switched to dextrose and water, because return of fluid to the bloodstream also means the return of salt.

How much fluid should be given? The amount depends on several things: the extent and depth of the patient's burns (which you must know how to estimate), his age, and past medical history. As you no doubt know, the correct amount will perfuse all organ systems and maintain normal blood pressure and urinary output without overloading the vascular system.

To accurately regulate—or titrate—the amount of fluid a burn patient like Karen should get, you closely monitor her output, as well as other vital signs. Generally, you figure fluid replacement is adequate when an adult's urinary output is from 30 to 60 ml/hour. For children or older patients, maintain an output from 10 to 30 ml/hour. (The doctor will probably order urinary output maintained at an even lower rate for children under age 4, patients over 60, and patients with respiratory problems.)

Caution: To reduce the risk of fluid overload, assess your patient frequently, and adjust the fluid rate, as needed.

Naturally, no rules exist to tell you *exactly* how much fluid to give each patient hourly. You must tailor titration to suit each patient. Consider Karen as an example. Her requirements will vary from hour to hour—depending on her condition—so you measure her intake and output frequently. She might need as much as 500 to 1000 ml of fluid per hour during the time she's in the E.D. Keep a close watch, using these guidelines to help you:

• Mark the I.V. bottle with tape to show hourly intake.

• Use a urine-measuring chamber—e.g., a urometer for the most accurate measurement of output.

CALCULATE EXTENT OF THE BURN

	Anterior	Posterior
head	_____	_____
neck	_____	_____
right arm	_____	_____
rt. forearm	_____	_____
right hand	_____	_____
left arm	_____	_____
lt. forearm	_____	_____
left hand	_____	_____
trunk	_____	_____
buttock	_____	_____
perineum	_____	_____
right thigh	_____	_____
right leg	_____	_____
right foot	_____	_____
left thigh	_____	_____
left leg	_____	_____
left foot	_____	_____
Subtotal	_____	_____
% TOTAL AREA BURNED	_____	

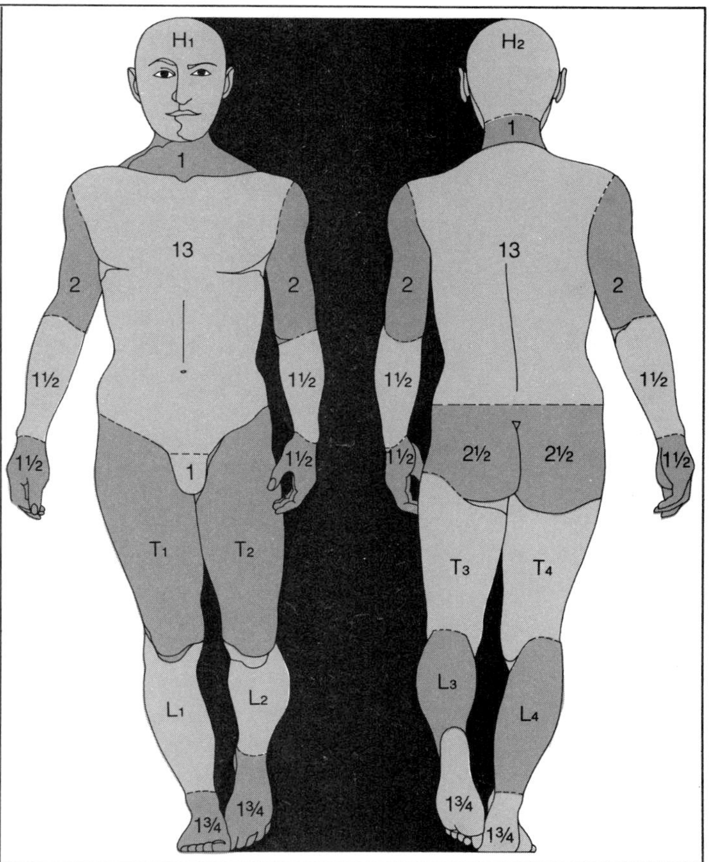

PATIENT'S AGE	0	1	5	10	15	Adult
H (1 or 2) = ½ of the head	9½	8½	6½	5½	4½	3½
T (1, 2, 3 or 4) = ½ of a thigh	2¾	3¼	4	4¼	4½	4¾
L (1, 2, 3 or 4) = ½ of a leg	2½	2½	2¾	3	3¼	3½

Evaluating burns

To calculate the extent of a patient's burn, follow these steps: 1) Shade the body diagrams above so they reflect the burn on each part of the patient's body, front and back. If only a portion of a body section is burned, shade only a portion of that area. 2) The numbers on the diagrams represent the percentage of the body that's burned. Record the numbers of the area you shade in the table above. If only a fraction of an area is burned, divide the number by that fraction, and record *that* number in the chart.

Remember that as children grow up, the proportions of their bodies change. These changes occur primarily in the head, thighs and legs, so the percentage of the body these areas represent varies according to age. Use the age table above to calculate the correct percentage for these areas. 3) Consider all parts of the body and then add the numbers to obtain a subtotal for anterior and posterior burns. Add these figures for the percentage of total body area burned. 4) When you gauge a burn's severity, consider the depth as well as the size. Consult the table on page 145 to assess the full extent of a burn.

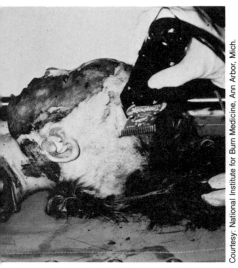

Courtesy: National Institute for Burn Medicine, Ann Arbor, Mich.

Wound care
To prevent infection in the severely burned patient, remove all hair from the burn wound and surrounding area, when he's admitted. If his scalp has been burned or if his hair lies near the wound, shave his scalp. Otherwise, trim his scalp hair to a 2″ length. Then shave a 2″ margin around all wounds.

- Never record an I.V. amount as infused until it actually *is* infused.
- If urine output increases over the previous hours, *slow* the I.V. rate
- If urine output decreases from the previous hours, *speed* the I.V. rate.
- Notify the doctor if Karen's urinary output exceeds or drops below the desired amount, or if she doesn't respond to the adjustments you've made in the flow rate within 1 hour.
- Make sure I.V. and urinary catheters remain patent. Check for a plugged urinary catheter if Karen's output falls.
- Weigh your patient and record the result on her chart. Later, nurses caring for Karen will use this figure as a baseline, because they'll expect a postadmission weight gain of up to 15% from burn shock and fluid therapy.

To guide titration, measure Karen's hematocrit on admission and every 6 to 8 hours during initial fluid replacement. Because water shifts from the bloodstream to the tissues during burn shock, the hematocrit starts high: Red blood cells are concentrated in relation to serum. With adequate fluid replacement, the hematocrit returns to normal. The patient may even become anemic a few days to a week postburn. This happens because the burn has damaged or destroyed red blood cells.

A very deep burn wound can immediately destroy many red blood cells and muscle tissue, releasing free hemoglobin and myoglobin into the bloodstream, where they'll be filtered out by the kidneys. These free globins may then plug the patient's kidney tubules, causing hemoglobinuria and impending renal failure. *Watch for black urine.* If you see it, tell the doctor at once. He'll want to flush Karen's kidneys by giving her an osmotic diuretic, such as mannitol, and temporarily increasing the I.V. flow rate to increase diuresis.

Other *stat* tests for the severely burned patient on admission are: electrolytes, CO_2 combining power, blood urea nitrogen (BUN), creatinine, serum protein level, blood type, and arterial blood-gas measurement. A chest X-ray is also taken.

Severe burns always put a strain on a patient's cardiovascular system, so make sure Karen has an EKG when she's admitted. Sometimes a patient's condition calls for repeated EKGs throughout therapy: for example, if a patient is over 60 or under 4, has an electrical burn, has congestive heart failure, or is taking reserpine or a digitalis glycoside.

What's in a burn?

Now let's get back to the burn wound. When a patient like Karen comes into the E.D., you'll have to clean her wounds—as well as her entire body—if you can't transport her to a specialized burn care facility within 3 to 4 hours. She'll probably have dirt and debris lodged in and around her wound because of the accident and, like most severely burned patients, she'll probably have loose, dead tissue on the burned area. If Karen was treated on the scene, someone may have put topical agents or dressings on her wounds. Of course, you'll remove these.

To simplify wound cleaning, immerse Karen in a hydrotherapy tub if you have one. Make sure the water is body temperature (99° F., 37.2° C.) and add a little surgical detergent, as well as enough salt to make it isotonic. If you can't put Karen in a tub, clean her wounds on an examining table, using a sterile saline-and-detergent solution and gauze squares.

Take care to clean burn wounds *gently;* never scrub burned skin with a brush. If you're not careful, you'll worsen tissue damage; for example, convert a partial-thickness burn to a full-thickness loss. (For a full discussion of the differences between the two types of burns, see page 145.)

As you wash Karen, look for carbon deposits deep in her wounds. *But don't try to dig them out.* Most of them will gradually come to the surface and get removed with dressing changes. One of the things you must do, however, is gently remove gross debris and any loose, sloughing skin. Snip away broken blisters with sterile forceps and scissors. Leave any blisters that aren't leaking untouched—even large ones. They're probably partial-thickness burns, and the blister serves as an ideal, naturally sterile dressing.

Shave any hairy area near or in the burn wound at this time, because hair harbors bacteria. Shave Karen's scalp if it's burned, or cut her hair very short (about 2″) if her scalp isn't burned. Always keep a razor and electric clippers on the emergency cart. Be sure to save Karen's hair for her family. They may want to keep it.

Apply dressings, as shown on page 153.

Does Karen have burns on her eyes, ears, hands, perineal area; or burns involving bone, muscle, or tendon? You need to give such wounds special attention when you clean them. Follow these guidelines:

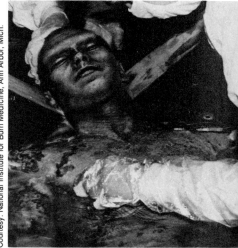

Courtesy: National Institute for Burn Medicine, Ann Arbor, Mich.

A vital soak
Hydrotherapy, or tubbing, promotes burn wound care in several ways. It reduces wound bacteria; it helps remove previously administered topical agents; it permits debridement of loose debris without trauma; it softens eschar, facilitating its removal; and it allows the patient to exercise his extremities with minimal friction.

Remember to rinse the patient's entire body as he leaves the tub. Never leave a burn patient unattended during hydrotherapy.

• *Eye care:* Gently clean area around eyes and lids with moistened applicators or gauze pads soaked in sterile solution. If the eyes or lids appear to be burned, soften and remove crusts, cover her eyes with saline-soaked pads, and call an eye doctor immediately.

• *Ear care:* Clip hair and shave a 2″ margin around the burned area. Clean out the external auditory canal with moistened applicators to remove crusts and debris. Protect the ear with moist dressings.

• *Nose care:* Cartilage and soft tissue within the nose can deteriorate quickly with infection. To minimize this risk, clean inside Karen's nostrils with moistened applicators to remove crusts and debris. If you've inserted a nasogastric tube, check that it's not taped too tightly.

• *Hand care:* Are Karen's fingers burned? Wrap each one with a separate, single-thickness of fine mesh gauze after cleaning—to prevent webbing. Keep the wrapping smooth: Don't let it fold or wrinkle. *Remember, burned surfaces should never touch each other.* Use this technique wherever two burned surfaces are apt to touch.

• *Perineal care:* Burn wounds in this area are at great risk of becoming contaminated. Clean and rinse them carefully, and put moist gauze dressings between burned buttocks.

• *Bone, muscle, and tendon care:* Has the burn wound exposed any of these? Don't permit them to dry. *Keep them moist at all times with dressings soaked in a sterile saline solution.*

Getting the patient ready to transport
As you've cleaned Karen's burn wounds, you've had a chance to evaluate them. By knowing what to look for, you can help the doctor greatly in his assessment. How serious Karen's burns are will determine where Karen should be treated and will predict her chance for survival. (Study page 145 for details on how to assess a burn's severity.)

Remember, most burns reveal a mixture of partial- and full-thickness damage to tissue. Because of this and the trauma of the accident, many patients need some pain medication for its sedative, as well as analgesic, effect. A word of caution, however. Give analgesics by I.V. only—not I.M—during the emergent period. The patient's hypotensive circulation may cause I.M. medication to pool and not be absorbed immediately. Then, when circulation returns to normal, the

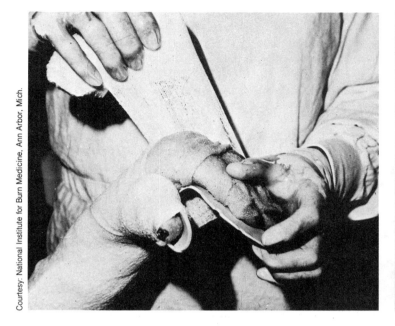

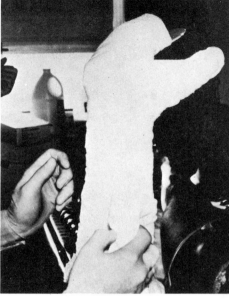

patient may absorb several doses at once and develop a toxic blood level.

Never give a pain medication like morphine to a patient when you anticipate respiratory problems. Morphine depresses respiration.

When wound care is complete, place Karen on a clean stretcher and cover her with a sterile sheet or bath blanket; the loss of protective skin cover makes chilling easy. Keep Karen warm by increasing the room temperature to over 75° F. (23.9° C.) or use a heat lamp. Continue to monitor her respiratory status, vital signs, and fluid titration until she's transferred.

Next, check to be sure Karen's care will be continued during transfer. Emphasize to transfer personnel the importance of keeping Karen's airway, I.V., and urinary catheter patent. Tell them to continue administering oxygen and to keep the nasogastric tube unclamped.

Don't forget emotional needs

Granted, emergency care for a severely burned patient like Karen can be hectic. But don't forget she is a person who needs your strong emotional support. Burn patients experi-

A helping hand
Splint palmar burns so that the fingers extend and the thumb abducts. To pad and protect the hand, first apply one layer of a fine-mesh gauze and one layer of Kerlix around palm and fingers. Then anchor the splint at the wrist so that the meta-carpophalangeal joints extend one inch beyond the bend in the splint. Wrap Kerlix around the entire hand to secure the splint in place.

ence excruciating mental stress from the shock of the accident, the pain, the chaos, and the rush to the hospital. Karen probably fears scarring and disfigurement. She needs you to be genuinely concerned for her welfare, and so does her anxious family.

You'll recall we said burns don't cause a patient to lose consciousness. Well, keep this in mind so you'll remember to talk to Karen. Tell her your name, and call her by hers so she can feel the comfort of contact with another human being. Orient her to her surroundings and prepare her, as well as you can, for what she can expect. Tell her about the equipment and procedures used during emergency care—and the reasons for them. Karen may be very unfamiliar with them, so she'll find them frightening.

Remember, too, that Karen's family needs help from the beginning. They're probably standing by waiting anxiously the whole time she's in the emergency department. Find a way to reassure them, if you can, and do your best to answer their questions. Suggest helpful ways that they might spend the necessary waiting time. Perhaps they'd like to go to the chapel or meet with the social worker.

What about your own emotional needs during this trying time? Nurses have feelings, too, of course. And the strain of treating a severely burned patient like Karen will leave you anxious and possibly upset. What's more, you'll probably react to the distress of her family, which—since her injury is life-threatening—will be very great indeed. Don't feel guilty if you experience anxiety and need emotional support. These feelings are normal for everyone working on the burn team.

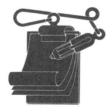

Remember these important points when caring for a patient with severe burns:
1. **Expect your patient to have breathing difficulties if he has face or neck burns, singed nasal hair, darkened sputum, and burn or carbon marks on his oral and nasal mucous membranes.**
2. **Remove clothing of the severely burned patient by cutting it along seam lines.**
3. **To determine the amount of fluid a burn patient needs, closely monitor output and other vital signs. Titrate fluids to each patient's needs.**
4. **Look for a dark, concentrated, decreased urine flow, which may indicate hemoglobinuria and impending renal failure.**

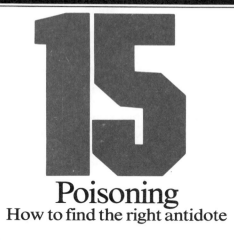

Poisoning
How to find the right antidote

MINNIE ROSE, RN, BSN, MEd

AT 5:45 P.M. ONE COLD WINTER EVENING, a station wagon pulls into the hospital parking lot, and 23-year-old Julia Wallace rushes her 4-year-old son, Mike, into the emergency department. She'd been preparing dinner when Mike, who was bored and hungry, emptied her purse and swallowed a large number of aspirin tablets. While another nurse tries to calm Mrs. Wallace and find out how many tablets Mike took, you assess his condition. He seems terrified; he's crying and hyperventilating. You have trouble keeping him still. According to Mrs. Wallace's estimates, Mike has swallowed approximately 30 aspirin tablets.

Prepare yourself now
Do you know what to do? What's the best method to rid Mike's system of the drug? Suppose he had swallowed something else? Or had been poisoned in another way? Would you be ready to make a quick, accurate assessment and to start appropriate treatment? This chapter will help you prepare for poison emergencies regardless of the route: ingestion, inhalation, or skin contamination. Learn what to do now while you have time. If you put it off, you may find you're too late.

Prevention pointers
The best precaution against
poisoning lies in patient
education. Here are some tips for
poison control to pass on to your
patient.
  • Read the label before you take
medicine.
  • Store all medications and
household chemicals properly.
Keep them out of the reach of
children.
  • Don't take medicines
prescribed for someone else.
  • Don't transfer medicines from
their original bottles to other
containers without labelling them
properly.
  • Don't take medications in the
dark or in front of small children.
  • Don't call medications
"candy" to make small children
take them.
  • Discard old medications.
  • Use toxic sprays only in
well-ventilated areas.
  • Wear a face mask and rubber
gloves when using pesticides.

The dangers of aspirin

Mike suffers from salicylate poisoning which kills more children under the age of five than any other accidental poisoning. An aspirin overdose stimulates the central nervous system and can cause tinnitus, vomiting, hyperventilation, fever, and hyperactivity. In severe cases — when a child absorbs more than 200 mg of aspirin per kilogram of body weight — he may also suffer convulsions, dehydration, decreased sensorium, respiratory failure, and cardiovascular collapse.

Let me explain why these symptoms occur. When Mike hyperventilates, he loses carbon dioxide. This loss causes respiratory alkalosis (an increased plasma pH). To compensate, his kidneys will excrete base in the form of bicarbonate, along with sodium, potassium, and organic acids. The patient may become dehydrated. The bodies of older children and adults usually stabilize at this point. However, in a very young child, you must watch carefully because the excessive loss of base from his system may overcorrect his condition and cause metabolic acidosis. Blood gas results may show a normal pH even though his PCO_2 will be below normal.

Treating an overdose

Knowing the danger Mike faces, what measures do you take? You already have recorded Mike's age, weight, the number of tablets he has swallowed, and the time he swallowed them — all vital information for his treatment. So your next step is to induce vomiting. To do this, you give Mike a tablespoon of syrup of ipecac followed by a glass of water. (If Mike were unconscious or convulsing, however, you would never induce vomiting since he might aspirate vomitus.)

Now start an I.V. of 5% dextrose in water, and draw arterial blood for measurement of blood gases and serum sodium, potassium, and salicylate levels. A serum salicylate level greater than 30 mg per 100 ml is usually toxic. Check Mike's vital signs, especially his respirations. If he develops a fever, give him a sponge bath with tepid water.

You can further increase the excretion of salicylates by alkalinizing Mike's urine (increasing the pH). Give sodium bicarbonate I.V. for this, but be careful: If you administer too much, you'll create severe alkalosis. Check Mike's plasma pH and urine pH closely. Watch for other signs of salicylate toxicity: proteinuria and an elevated serum amylase.

The doctor may also order gastric lavage for Mike. If so, instill 30 ml of fluid at a time, aspirate the stomach contents, and then repeat until the returns are clear. Save vomitus and aspirated stomach contents for analysis.

Since some doctors feel that gastric lavage only helps salicylates dissolve faster, you may be told to use activated charcoal to inactivate the poison. If so, instill through the nasogastric tube a solution of one or two tablespoons of activated charcoal mixed in a glass of water. If the patient is conscious, give him activated charcoal only after you've made him vomit with ipecac. Otherwise the charcoal will inactivate the syrup of ipecac if given prior to emptying the stomach. Remember to lower a lethargic patient's head so he doesn't aspirate the stomach contents. To avoid this problem, the doctor may insert a cuffed endotracheal tube before lavage.

If several hours have passed since the patient ingested the overdose, use large quantities of I.V. fluids to flush his kidneys. The kind of fluid you'll use depends upon the patient's acid/base balance. Remember that acidosis can cause a toxic shift of salicylates from the plasma into the brain tissue. For this reason the doctor may order sodium bicarbonate added to the I.V. fluids. The recommended dose (2 to 5 mEq/kg) for adults and older children is to be given over 4 to 8 hours.

To promote diuresis, the doctor may also order 250 mg of acetazolamide (Diamox) daily for 1 to 2 days, or mannitol, 5% to 10% solutions (500 to 1000 ml) to be infused continuously until the patient can maintain a urine flow of 100 ml/hour. Monitor the intake and output carefully; remember that the patient shouldn't receive more than 200 grams (2000 ml of a 10% solution) in a 24-hour period.

Once diuresis is assured, the doctor may have you add potassium to the I.V. solution. The dosage is adjusted to the patient's needs. But the usual dose for adults and older children is 2 mEq/kg of body weight of potassium for 12 hours, the total not to exceed 20 mEq/L. Of course, for a child under 12, the doctor will calculate a smaller, appropriate dose.

Since Mike swallowed the aspirin only a short time ago, chances are he may not need any treatment beyond emesis. Of course, since aspirin will take 48 hours to move through his body, he should be hospitalized for observation during that period.

What about cases that involve substances other than aspi-

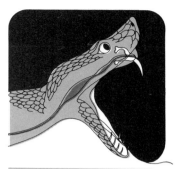

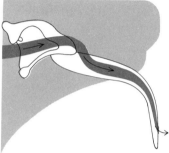

Snake in the grass?
Poisonous snakes inhabit every state in the United States except Hawaii, Alaska, and Maine. Even though snakebite victims represent a small percentage of E.D. cases, be prepared to act quickly in such an emergency.

The snake pictured above is a rattlesnake. When it bites its victim, the contracting muscles squeeze venom from a gland in each cheek along a hollow tube within the fang and out the tip.

Snakebite victims commonly arrive at the E.D. with a tourniquet tied tightly around the affected extremity. If so, don't remove the tourniquet as this would release the venom suddenly into the patient's system.

Call the doctor, maintain a patent airway, and begin I.V. fluids. The doctor will prescribe antivenin and oxygen. Keep the patient quiet and the affected part immobile.

**National
Poison Center
Network®
Poison Treatment Chart**

How to use this chart

Locate the substance that has poisoned your patient in the columns to the right. The number listed after the poison corresponds with the appropriate treatment in the management column below.

Suggested general treatment for poisoning management

1. There should be no problem in small amounts.
   No treatment necessary.
   Fluids may be given.
2. Induce vomiting. Give Syrup of Ipecac in the following dosages:
   Under one year of age:
   Two teaspoons followed by at least 2-3 glasses of liquid.
   One year and over:
   Give one tablespoon followed by at least 2-3 glasses of liquid.
   Do not induce vomiting if the patient is semicomatose, comatose, or convulsing.
   Call Poison Center for additional information.
3. Dilute or neutralize with water or milk. **Do not induce vomiting.** Gastric lavage is indicated. Call Poison Center for specific instructions.
4. Treat symptomatically unless botulism is suspected. Call Poison Center for specific information regarding botulism.
5. Dilute or neutralize with water or milk. **Do not induce vomiting.** Gastric lavage should be avoided. This substance may cause burns of the mucous membranes. Consult E.N.T. specialist following emergency treatment. Call Poison Center for specific information.
6. Immediately wash skin thoroughly with running water. Call Poison Center for further treatment.
7. Immediately wash eyes with a gentle stream of running water. Continue for 15 minutes. Call Poison Center for further treatment.
8. Specific antagonist may be indicated. Call Poison Center.
9. Remove to fresh air. Support respirations. Call Poison Center for further treatment.
10. Call Poison Center for specific instructions.
11. Symptomatic and supportive treatment. **Do not induce vomiting** for ingestions. I.V. Naloxone Hydrochloride (Narcan) to be given as indicated for respiratory depression.
    Dosage:
    Adult — 0.4 mg I.V.
    May be repeated at 2-3 min. intervals.
    Child — 0.01 mg/kg I.V.
    May be repeated at 5-10 min. intervals.

A

Acetone 2
Acids
   Ingestion 5
   Eye Contamination 7
   Topical 6
   Inhalation if mixed with bleach
  9
Aerosols
   Eye Contamination 7
   Inhalation 9
After Shave Lotions See Cologne
Airplane Glue 10
Alcohol
   Ingestion 2
   Eye Contamination 7
Ammonia
   Ingestion 5
   Eye Contamination 7
   Inhalation 9
Amphetamine 2, 8
Analgesics 10
Aniline Dyes
   Ingestion 2, 8
   Inhalation 8, 9
   Topical 6, 8
Antacids 1
Antibiotics
   Less than 2-3 times total
   daily dose 1
   More than 3 times total
   daily dose 2
Antidepressants
   Tricyclic 2, 8
   Others 2
Antifreeze (Ethylene Glycol)
   Ingestion 2
   Eye Contamination 7
Antihistamines 2, 8
Antiseptics 2
Ant Trap: Kepone Type 1
             Others 2
Aquarium Products 1
Arsenic 2, 8
Aspirin 2

B

Baby Oil 1
Ball Point Ink 1
Barbiturates
   Short Acting 10
   Long Acting 2
Bathroom Bowl Cleaner
   Ingestion 5
   Eye Contamination 7
   Inhalation if mixed with bleach
  9
   Topical 6
Batteries
   Dry Cell (Flash Light) 1
   Mercury (Hearing Aid) 2
   Wet Cell (Automobile) 5
Benzene
   Ingestion 10

   Inhalation 9
   Topical 6
Birth Control Pills 1
Bleaches
   Liquid Ingestion 1
   Solid Ingestion 5
   Eye Contamination 7
   Inhalation when mixed with
   acids or alkalies 9
Boric Acid 2
Bromides 2
Bubble Bath 1

C

Camphor 2
Candles 1
Caps
   Less than One Roll 1
   More than One Roll 2
Carbon Monoxide 9
Carbon Tetrachloride
   Ingestion 2
   Inhalation 9
   Topical 6
Chalk 1
Chlorine Bleach . .See Bleaches
Cigarettes
   Less than One 1
   One or More 2
Clay .1
Cleaning Fluids 10
Cleanser (household) 1
Clinitest Tablets 5
Cold Remedies 10
Cologne
   Less than 15cc 1
   More than 15cc 2
Contraceptive Pills 1
Corn-Wart Removers 5
Cosmetics . . .See Specific Type
Cough Medicines 10
Crayons
   Children's 1
   Others 2
Cyanide 8

D

Dandruff Shampoo 2
Dehumidifying Packets 1
Denture Adhesives 1
Denture Cleansers 5
Deodorants
   All Types 1
Deodorizer Cakes 2
Deodorizers, Room 10
Desiccants 1
Detergents
   Liquid-Powder (General) . . .1
   Electric Dishwasher and
   Phosphate Free 5
Diaper Rash Ointment 1
Dishwasher
   Detergents . . .See Detergents
Disinfectants 3
Drain Cleaners . . . . .See Lye

Courtesy: Richard W. Moriarty, MD, Director, National Poison Center Network, Children's Hospital of Pittsburgh

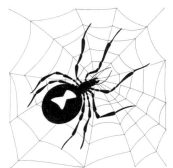

Along came a spider
Black widow spider bites may go
unnoticed until severe pain at the
puncture site and intense
cramping abdominal pain strike
the victim 10-40 minutes later.
Since no lab test can detect the
cause, a diagnosis must be made
clinically. When taking a history,
ask the patient if he's recently
been in a lumber or junk pile, an
outdoor privy, or an old barn,
garage or basement. Black widow
spiders may inhabit any of these
places.

Here's how to recognize and
treat symptoms of spider bites.

Spider bite victims may suffer
spasmodic muscle pain in the
legs, chest and back. At the
puncture site you'll see two tiny
red spots and slight swelling or
urticaria. The patient will
experience weakness, nausea,
fever, chills, and a rigid abdomen
with diminished bowel sounds.
He'll have elevated blood
pressure, labored breathing,
profuse sweating, and numb or
tingling feet. Small children may
suffer delirium and convulsions.

Keep the patient quiet and the
affected part immobile. If a
tourniquet is in place, check his
pulse regularly. Don't release the
tourniquet as this would also
release toxins into the circulatory
system. Apply cold packs to
relieve pain and swelling and to
slow circulation.

rin? Always ask a family member or the patient himself, if you can, what he swallowed, when, and how much. Make sure you know the patient's age and weight. If the poison came in a bottle, ask what was on the label and have the container brought to the hospital, if possible. *Nursing tip:* If you don't know what substance the patient has swallowed, look for burns in and around his mouth, smell his breath for any unusual odors, and examine his hands and clothing for stains or residue. *Do not induce emesis if the patient swallowed any petroleum products or corrosive acids since they would further burn his digestive tract if vomited.*

Use the chart on page 158-159 to find the appropriate treatment for many poisons. And remember: *You and every other nurse in your unit should know the phone number of the Poison Control Center in your area.*

Poisons in the air
Not all poisoning cases involve ingestion, of course. Patients who were exposed to dangerous gases such as chlorine, carbon dioxide, hydrogen sulfide, nitrogen dioxide, and ammonia usually need emergency care in the hospital. This is because gas poisoning can cause frank respiratory distress. The extent of damage depends on how soluble the gas is. The more soluble gases will irritate a patient's upper respiratory tract, but usually won't cause lasting damage if he is able to leave the contaminated area quickly. Less soluble gases, like nitrogen dioxide, irritate the patient's lower respiratory tract. Since he won't cough or gag from the fumes, he probably won't notice any signs of poisoning until he's developed severe bronchiolitis and pulmonary edema.

To illustrate what I'm talking about, let's consider the following case. One night when you are on duty in the E.D., the ambulance brings in several patients who were poisoned by chlorine gas leaking from a nearby water treatment plant. You care for Jeffrey Saunders, age 29, who coughs, wheezes, and has great difficulty breathing. His eyes tear, and he moans and complains of severe burning in his throat.

Immediately place Mr. Saunders in a semi-Fowler's position and start oxygen by mask at 6 liters per minute. Then, start an I.V. of 5% dextrose in water. In this case, Mr. Saunders responds quickly to the treatment. He's admitted to the hospital for observation where he starts on a bronchodilator

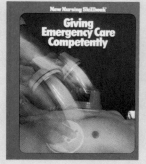
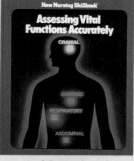
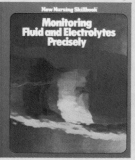
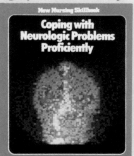
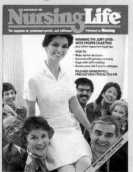

Get to know the NEW NURSING SKILLBOOK series. Examine your first—and every volume—free before you buy.

- Coping With Neurologic Problems Proficiently
- Managing Diabetics Properly
- Monitoring Fluid and Electrolytes Precisely
- Giving Cardiovascular Drugs Safely
- Assessing Vital Functions Accurately
- Nursing Critically Ill Patients Confidently
- Giving Emergency Care Competently
- Reading EKGs Correctly
- Combatting Cardiovascular Diseases Skillfully
- Dealing with Death and Dying

Each NEW NURSING SKILLBOOK gives you ● **skillchecks** ● **complete indexing** ● **easy-to-follow text that makes everything plain** ● **clear illustrations** ● **a quality hardcover binding.**

Send this postage-paid card to get your first copy of *NursingLife*.

NO-RISK, MONEY-BACK GUARANTEE

If you're not delighted with your first issue of *NursingLife*, simply write "cancel" across your bill. You won't be charged a cent. And if at *any* time you feel *NursingLife* isn't helping you enough, cancel your subscription. You'll promptly get a refund for the unmailed issues. So order today!

What's for dinner?

Food poisoning causes acute illness and requires aggressive treatment. A patient may become sick by accidentally ingesting poisonous plants (see pages 162 and 163), or by eating food that's been chemically contaminated, or, most commonly, by eating food contaminated by bacteria. The table below describes this third form of food poisoning.

If many people are stricken after ingesting the same tainted food, a doctor can diagnose food poisoning fairly easily. But if only one person becomes ill, diagnosing him may be more difficult. Testing a sample of the suspected food in the laboratory may confirm food poisoning.

Remember not to administer anti-diarrheals during the first 24 hours after the patient ingests the contaminated food, unless it's absolutely necessary. Diarrhea helps rid the body of the toxin and is a natural response to poisoning. Above all, give the patient strong emotional support. He'll feel extremely ill and your care can make him less anxious.

DISEASES CAUSED BY MICROORGANISMS OR THEIR TOXINS

ORGANISM	FOOD	SYMPTOMS	DIAGNOSTIC TEST	TREATMENT
Clostridium botulinum	Inadequately processed vegetables and meat	Nausea and vomiting, abdominal pain, weakness, dry mouth, dizziness, blurred vision, diplopia, dysphagia, dysarthria	Examination of suspected food, or of vomitus and feces for C. botulinum	Cathartics, emesis, gastric lavage, polyvalent botulism antitoxin; respiratory support, non-narcotic sedative
Clostridium perfringens	Cold or rewarmed meats and gravy	Griping abdominal pain, diarrhea nausea and vomiting (usually mild gastroenteritis)	Anaerobic culture of food	Symptomatic treatment, antispasmodics, non-narcotic analgesics or sedatives
Salmonella non-typhoidal	Water, poultry, eggs, egg products, dried foods and wild animal meat	Abrupt onset of colicky abdominal pain, nausea and vomiting, diarrhea, fever	Culture of feces and blood; isolation of one of the types of Salmonella	Symptomatic treatment, antispasmodics, fluid and electrolyte replacement; bland diet
Shigella	Food contaminated by feces of infected persons	Fever, abdominal pain, bloody diarrhea	Culture of feces, isolation of Shigella from the stools (sometimes low plasma CO_2 is found, reflecting diarrhea-induced metabolic acidosis)	Fluid and electrolyte replacement; Tetracycline, 2.5 grams as a single adult oral dose or ampicillin, 50 mg per kg/day for 5 days; analgesics
Staphylococcus aureus	Meat, dairy products	Nausea and vomiting, abdominal pain, diarrhea; in some cases fever and headache	Gram stain and culture of suspected food for coagulase-positive staphylococci	Symptomatic treatment; rapid I.V. fluid replacement, if necessary

Plant chart key
The colored area on these pages indicates the poisonous part of the plant. In cases where the poisonous part could not be pictured, it is listed in parentheses after the plant name.

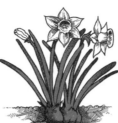

DAFFODIL
Sx: GI distress and convulsions
Rx: gastric lavage or emesis; symptomatic treatment

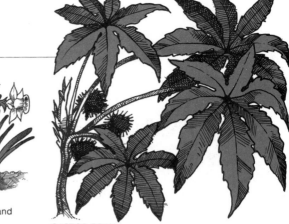

CASTOR BEAN
Sx: GI distress, burning throat, thirst, convulsions
Rx: gastric lavage or emesis; sodium bicarbonate

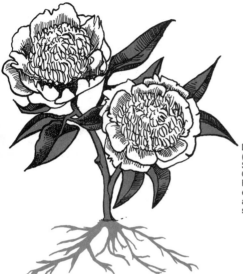

PEONY (roots)
Sx: paralysis, GI distress, convulsions
Rx: gastric lavage or emesis; mannitol, symptomatic treatment

DIEFFENBACHIA
(dumbcane)
Sx: burning throat, edema, GI distress
Rx: gastric lavage or emesis; antihistamines and lime juice; symptomatic treatment

NARCISSUS
Sx: GI distress and convulsions
Rx: gastric lavage or emesis; symptomatic treatment

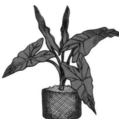

ELEPHANT EAR PHILODENDRON
Sx: burning throat and GI distress
Rx: gastric lavage or emesis; antihistamines and lime juice; symptomatic treatment

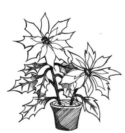

POINSETTIA (milky juice)
Sx: inflammation and blisters
Rx: none; condition will disappear after several days

POTATO (green, spoiled, sprouted)
Sx: GI distress, CNS disturbances, shock
Rx: gastric lavage or emesis; symptomatic treatment, respiratory support, paraldehyde

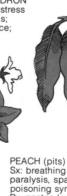

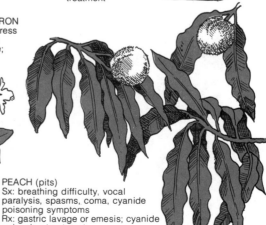

PEACH (pits)
Sx: breathing difficulty, vocal paralysis, spasms, coma, cyanide poisoning symptoms
Rx: gastric lavage or emesis; cyanide poisoning treatment

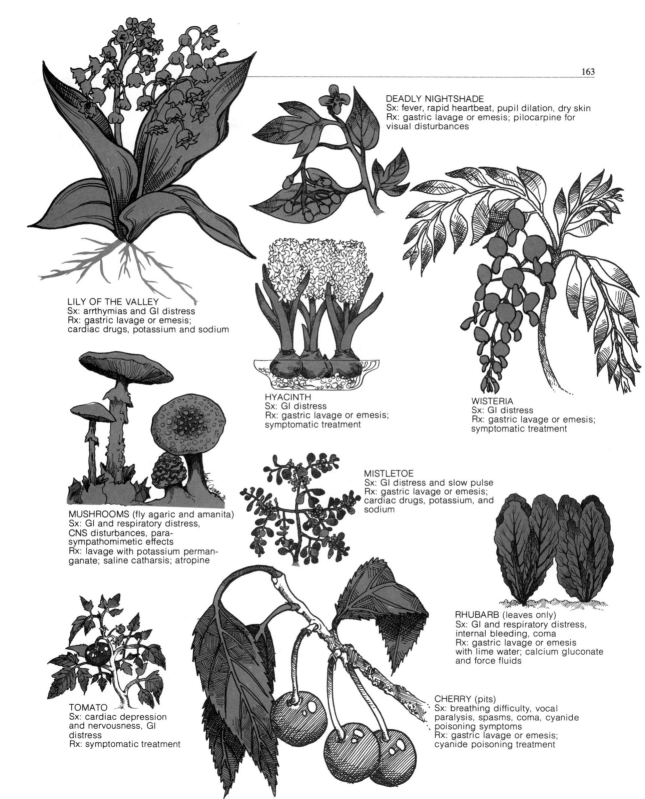

163

DEADLY NIGHTSHADE
Sx: fever, rapid heartbeat, pupil dilation, dry skin
Rx: gastric lavage or emesis; pilocarpine for
visual disturbances

LILY OF THE VALLEY
Sx: arrthymias and GI distress
Rx: gastric lavage or emesis;
cardiac drugs, potassium and sodium

HYACINTH
Sx: GI distress
Rx: gastric lavage or emesis;
symptomatic treatment

WISTERIA
Sx: GI distress
Rx: gastric lavage or emesis;
symptomatic treatment

MUSHROOMS (fly agaric and amanita)
Sx: GI and respiratory distress,
CNS disturbances, para-
sympathomimetic effects
Rx: lavage with potassium perman-
ganate; saline catharsis; atropine

MISTLETOE
Sx: GI distress and slow pulse
Rx: gastric lavage or emesis;
cardiac drugs, potassium, and
sodium

RHUBARB (leaves only)
Sx: GI and respiratory distress,
internal bleeding, coma
Rx: gastric lavage or emesis
with lime water; calcium gluconate
and force fluids

TOMATO
Sx: cardiac depression
and nervousness, GI
distress
Rx: symptomatic treatment

CHERRY (pits)
Sx: breathing difficulty, vocal
paralysis, spasms, coma, cyanide
poisoning symptoms
Rx: gastric lavage or emesis;
cyanide poisoning treatment

after he receives an anitbiotic to prevent bronchitis. *Nursing tip:* When you're giving emergency care for gas poisoning, always alert the anesthesia department and have plenty of oxygen on hand. Some patients may require intubation.

Skin contamination

Some chemicals produce toxic effects when absorbed through the skin: for example, aniline dyes, chlordane, mercury, nicotine, phenol, thallium, parathion, and boric acid.

For example, when boric acid is used indiscriminately to treat an infant's diaper rash or eczema, it can cause abdominal distress, anorexia, erythema, headache, restlessness, and weakness. In severe cases—which can be fatal—infants may also develop tachycardia, kidney damage, convulsions, and circulatory collapse. *Nursing tip:* To treat boric acid poisoning, wash the patient's skin immediately with water. For severe cases, the doctor may prescribe oxygen, I.V. fluids, blood transfusions, and anticonvulsants.

Occasionally, you may see a patient who's used an insecticide recklessly, spilling the dangerous chemicals on his skin. For example, liquid parathion, an organic phosphate, is rapidly absorbed by all routes. A victim of parathion poisoning usually comes to the E.D. with local muscarinic-like effects: swelling, local contraction of the muscle, eye irritation, excessive salivation, sweating, miosis, and respiratory distress.

When you care for a patient with skin-contamination poisoning, make sure he has a patent airway. Then wash the skin thoroughly and start an I.V. of 5% dextrose in water.

To counteract the muscarinic-like effects, the doctor usually prescribes 2 to 4 mg of atropine I.V., repeating a 2-mg dose every 3 to 10 minutes until the symptoms disappear.

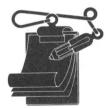

Remember these important points when caring for a patient after poisoning:
1. Give a conscious patient activated charcoal only after you've made him vomit with ipecac.
2. Increase salicylate excretion by alkalizing the patient's urine with sodium bicarbonate.
3. Ask the patient or a family member what was swallowed, when, how much, and if they still have the container.
4. Do not administer antidiarrheals during the first 24 hours after a patient ingests contaminated food, unless necessary.

16

Anaphylactic Shock
How to reverse a deadly reaction

BARBARA F. McVAN, RN

YOUR SHIFT HAS been hectic, but it's almost over. You've just sent a police officer to the operating room for repair of an abdominal gunshot wound. A half hour earlier, a letter carrier was transferred in stable condition to the CCU after being treated for myocardial infarction. Sandwiched between these major emergencies were three others: a 78-year-old woman with a fractured right arm, a 3-year-old with a concussion, and a teenager in insulin shock.

Now you're assisting the doctor as he sutures the lacerated hand of an auto mechanic. Suddenly, the receptionist tells you over the intercom that Doug Campbell, a phone company lineman, has just come to the emergency department with a bee sting on the left hand.

Does a bee sting require emergency care?
What do you do? Should you classify Mr. Campbell's bee sting as a real emergency? Could he go into anaphylactic shock? If he did, would you recognize the symptoms? What emergency care must you give a patient with this type of shock? His life may depend on your skills. That's why we've included this chapter to help you deal with this crisis effectively.

Identifying the high-risk patient

Let's get back to Mr. Campbell. How likely is he to develop anaphylactic shock? If you can't leave the patient you're caring for at that moment, ask the receptionist to ask him the following questions:

• "Have you ever been stung by an insect before?"

• "Have you ever had a reaction to an insect sting? If so, what type of reaction? Describe it in detail."

• "Are you under a doctor's care for any other disorders: for example, a respiratory condition, such as emphysema or asthma?"

• "Are you having any difficulty breathing since the sting? Does your chest feel tight? Do you itch? Have you noticed any swelling other than that around the sting?"

As soon as the receptionist gets the answers to these questions from the patient, have her give you the information. If he has a history of severe allergic reactions, or shows any of the following symptoms, he needs help immediately. Watch for:

• *respiratory distress* (dyspnea, wheezing, choking, and cyanosis)

• *dermatologic changes* (urticaria, erythema, angioedema, and pruritis)

• *gastrointestinal complaints* (nausea, vomiting, abdominal cramps, and diarrhea)

• *vascular collapse* (rapidly falling blood pressure, sweating, weakness, anxiety, dizziness, and thready pulse).

What causes anaphylactic shock?

Anaphylactic shock is a severe and deadly systemic reaction that can occur when a person comes in contact with an antigen to which he's acutely sensitive. Common antigens that may trigger anaphylactic shock include drugs (such as penicillin or those containing horse serum), venom from stinging insects (such as bee, wasp, or hornet), and diagnostic dyes.

Severe symptoms develop swiftly, and death can occur within minutes if the condition is left untreated. Work quickly when you suspect anaphylactic shock. The faster a patient's symptoms develop, the more likely he is to die.

Priorities for care

Depending on the patient's condition, the doctor will want you to follow these guidelines:

• Check for an open airway by assessing the patient's breathing, as described in Chapter 3. Watch closely for signs of respiratory distress. He may develop sudden airway obstruction from laryngeal edema. If this happens, be ready to give mouth-to-mouth resuscitation or insert an oral airway and apply mechanical ventilation. Keep an emergency tray handy in case the doctor has to perform a tracheostomy. Endotracheal intubation is usually difficult when laryngeal edema exists.

• Administer epinephrine (Adrenalin) 0.3 to 0.5 ml I.M., I.V., or subcutaneously; vigorously massage the injection site to increase absorption. Repeat the dose every 3 to 5 minutes, administering four or five doses. Epinephrine has a rapid antagonist effect on histamine; it acts as a bronchodilator and increases blood pressure by vasoconstriction. In many cases, this drug may produce a complete reversal of the patient's symptoms.

• Administer an antihistamine, such as diphenhydramine (Benadryl), 50 to 100 mg orally, I.M., or I.V. (depending on the patient's condition, size, and age). As you know, an antihistamine like Benadryl will not prevent histamine release or neutralize circulating histamine. But it will compete with released histamine at the receptor binding sites and block further absorption. This drug, given in combination with epinephrine, may be the only treatment the patient requires.

• If shock symptoms continue, start an I.V. with lactated Ringer's solution, using a large-bore catheter. Fluid administration supports the patient's jeopardized circulatory system. The large-bore catheter makes it easier to give needed medications intravenously.

• If epinephrine fails to control the patient's anaphylaxis, administer a vasopresser, such as norepinephrine injection (Levophed), by I.V. infusion to constrict the vessels. The recommended dosage is 8 to 12 mcg/minute initially, then 2 to 4 mcg/minute. *Caution:* Check the patient's blood pressure at regular intervals, and watch the injection site carefully for signs of drug infiltration: redness and swelling. Tissue infiltration can cause necrosis.

Depending on the severity of the reaction, the doctor may also order:

• dexamethasone (Decadron) to maintain blood pressure and prevent further systemic reactions. The recommended dosage for cases of anaphylactic shock is 4 mg bolus given *stat,* then 12 mg by I.V. infusion, administered slowly.

• Aminophylline to combat bronchospasms and alleviate asthma symptoms. The usual dosage for adults is 500 mg orally or by suppository immediately, and then 250 to 500 mg every 6 to 8 hours. Children should receive 7.5 mg/kg immediately, then 3 to 6 mg/kg every 6 to 8 hours.

When the patient recovers

Fortunately, you can almost always reverse anaphylactic shock with prompt, effective action. But your responsibility doesn't end there. Your patient must be taught how important it is for him to avoid future contact with the affecting antigen.

If his occupation makes this impossible, urge him to talk to the doctor about desensitization injections. Explain how these injections can help; warn him how dangerous it may be to do without them. *Nursing tip:* Desensitization injections should always be given under an allergist's supervision. If you ever are ordered to administer them, keep emergency drugs and equipment nearby in case of an adverse reaction.

Tell the patient to carry identification that will advise others of his potential for severe allergic reaction. For example, you might suggest Medic-Alert jewelry, which is readily available in most drugstores.

If you're caring for a patient who risks severe reaction from insect stings or other antigens, the doctor may give him an emergency kit, such as the one shown on the opposite page. Find out how the doctor has instructed him to use it. Then, reinforce his teaching by explaining how to give an injection and answering any questions the patient may have about the contents of the kit. To help you teach the patient how to use his kit, which includes a tourniquet, you may copy the patient teaching aid shown on the opposite page.

An additional reminder: A patient who has received medications for anaphylactic shock may still experience side effects from these medications after he's left the hospital. Be sure to warn him about these side effects. For example, epinephrine may cause rapid heartbeat in some patients, depending on the dosage given; antihistamines may cause drowsiness and dizziness.

Make prevention your responsibility

Remember, you have a major responsibility for preventing

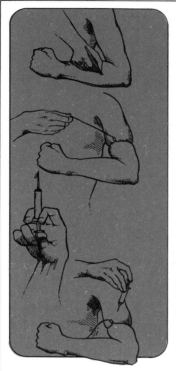

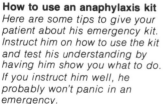

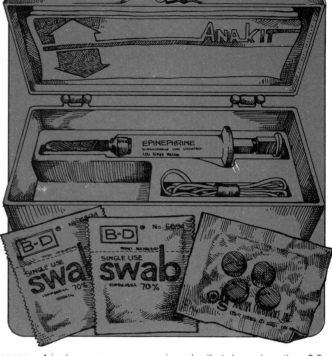

How to use an anaphylaxis kit

Here are some tips to give your patient about his emergency kit. Instruct him on how to use the kit and test his understanding by having him show you what to do. If you instruct him well, he probably won't panic in an emergency.

1. Contact doctor if possible, then proceed with emergency kit.
2. Remove insect stinger if it's still there. Don't push, pinch, squeeze, or further imbed stinger into skin.
3. If you were stung on an arm or leg, apply tourniquet between sting and body. To tighten, pull end of one string. Release tourniquet every 10 minutes by pulling metal ring.
4. Using an alcohol swab, cleanse a 4-inch area on arm or thigh (above tourniquet).
5. Prepare prefilled syringe. First, remove needle cover. Then, expel air from syringe by holding syringe with needle pointing up and carefully pushing plunger.
6. Inject epinephrine. Insert whole needle straight down into cleansed skin area. When this is done, pull back on plunger. If blood enters syringe, the needle is in a blood vessel. Withdraw needle, and reinsert in another site. For adults and children over 12 years, push plunger until it stops (0.3 cc). Do not force further. Replace needle cover. A second injection of 0.3 cc remains in syringe. Children 12 years and younger: H-S Epinephrine 1:1000 syringe has graduations of 0.1 cc

in order that doses less than 0.3 cc can be measured. Infants to 2 years: 0.05-0.1 cc; 2-6 years: 0.15 cc; 6-12 years: 0.2 cc.
7. Chew and swallow Chol-amine (antihistamine). Adults and children over 12 years should take 4 tablets; children 12 years or younger should take 2 tablets.
8. Apply ice packs if available.
9. Keep warm. Avoid exertion.
10. Prepare prefilled syringe for second injection. Turn rectangular plunger ¼ turn to right to line up with rectangular slot in syringe. Do not depress plunger until ready for second injection.
11. Second injection: If no noticeable improvement in 10 minutes, repeat steps 4, 5, and 6.
12. See doctor as soon as possible.

certain allergic reactions in your patients. This is especially true when the patient has an acute sensitivity to a particular drug or diagnostic dye.

Getting an adequate patient history during your initial interview will help you. Know what questions to ask and how to ask them. For example, don't just ask the patient if he has any allergies. Ask him if he's allergic to any drug, and if he says "Yes," ask him what kind of reaction he's had to it. A patient may not understand what an allergic reaction is. He may think the doctor no longer gives him a particular drug for that reason, when the doctor really switched drugs to effect a better cure.

Don't forget to ask the patient if he's allergic to any foods, insect stings, or inhalants when you take his history. If he has hay fever and comes to the hospital for surgery in late August or early September, you may think he's developed postoperative pneumonia, when he's only suffering his usual reaction to plant pollens. *Caution:* Never rely on a chart, Kardex, color-coded bracelet, or sign above the patient's bed to alert you to his allergies. Before you give any medication—in the hospital or in a clinic—always identify the drug and ask the patient if he's taken it before. Lethal drug errors have resulted because an allergy warning wasn't posted where the nurse looked for it. Never assume the patient has no allergy before you give a drug; always ask him.

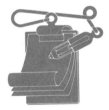

Remember these important points when caring for a patient in anaphylactic shock:
1. If the patient has a history of severe allergic reaction, respiratory distress, dermatologic changes, gastrointestinal complaints, or vascular collapse, consider the possibility of anaphylactic shock and take immediate action.
2. Act quickly when you suspect anaphylactic shock. When left untreated, death can occur within minutes.
3. Administer epinephrine (Adrenalin) 0.3 to 0.5 ml I.M., I.V., or subcutaneously, as ordered.
4. Advise the patient to carry identification (such as a Medi-Alert necklace or bracelet) that will alert others to his potential for a severe allergic reaction.
5. When taking a patient history, be sure to ask open-ended questions, such as "Do you have a reaction when you take any drugs?"

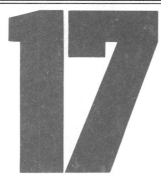

Psychiatric Emergencies
When stress gets the upper hand

PEGGY ELEANOR GORDON, RN, BSN, MSN
AND EILEEN NOTE, RN, BSN, MSN

THROUGHOUT THIS BOOK, you've heard about the physical problems that can bring a patient in for emergency care — but nothing's been said about the psychiatric problems. Especially those than can result from a stress: namely, agitation, confusion, and depression.

A patient may come in with any of these conditions, or one may develop during his treatment for something else. Would you know what to do for a patient displaying such abnormal behavior? Would you know what *not* to do?

Classify agitation, confusion, and depression as emergencies when you see them — for these reasons:

• agitation, because it can cause a patient to hurt himself or others

• confusion, because it can render a patient totally incompetent, and may be caused by a serious organic problem

• depression, because it can lead a patient to suicide.

Agitation: Easy to recognize
Let's consider agitation; it's easy to recognize. You can spot it quickly in a patient who wrings his hands, paces, bites his nails, talks incessantly, twitches, grimaces, shakes, swings his

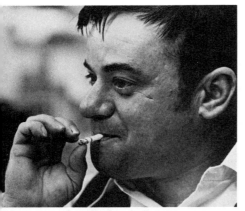

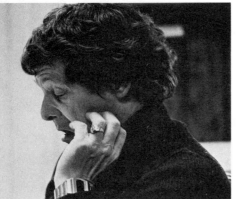

Coping with stress
The problem that brings a patient into an emergency department generally causes him great stress. His situation may not provide an outlet for his emotions, so his nervousness will be reflected in his body language, as shown in the illustrations on these two pages. By observing him carefully, you can tell a great deal about his mental state. This will help you anticipate his behavior and identify his needs.

legs, or repeats some purposeless action ritualistically.

Such a person can't sit still, concentrate, or complete any task; in fact, he may even be assaultive. Typically, the agitated person also shows physiologic hyperactivity: tachycardia, hyperventilation, gastrointestinal distress, urinary frequency, headaches, and other somatic disorders.

Such obvious agitation seems easy to recognize but doesn't always tell the whole story. A seemingly agitated person may, in fact, be suffering a severe underlying depression or organic disease. Agitation can also develop in any patient under stress. What happened to 16-year-old Susan Murray is not unusual.

Susan was brought to our emergency department with only superficial lacerations, after an automobile accident in which her boyfriend died instantly. At first, she was calm and cooperative, but later—when the doctor was about to discharge her—she became very upset.

"It's all my fault Johnny died," she screamed hysterically, and tried to run out the door.

We kept her from doing this, by sitting her down and speaking to her calmly. But Susan couldn't relax, nor would she accept our reassurance. Indeed, she seemed not to hear anything we said to her; she just kept jumping up and screaming about her boyfriend.

Susan needed a sedative to help her cope with her anguish, so we gave her diazepam (Valium) I.V., as the doctor ordered. And of course, we stayed with her while the medication took effect. In about 15 minutes, Susan calmed down and began to weep quietly—an appropriate response to the tragedy she faced. She was once again in control of herself and later returned home to her parents.

What causes agitation? Anxiety, depression, drug and alcohol intoxication and withdrawal, organic brain disease, and psychosis. And some patients whose problems are mostly physical can become agitated from fear and anxiety. For example, hospitalized patients may see themselves as helpless and dependent—they have lost some control over what is done to them, and, to add to their distress, they may fear the outcome of their hospitalization. To release the cumulative tensions that these fears create, the patient sometimes explodes into agitated behavior. Keep in mind that such behavior usually responds to simple reassurance and does not reflect a true psychotic state.

Coping: More difficult

Much more difficult than recognizing agitation is coping with it in a helpful way. Perhaps the most difficult part is coping with your own feelings toward the agitated person, particularly if he's assaultive. Then you have to overcome your fear which, under the circumstances, is understandable. Remember, too, that agitated persons are hard to redirect, so you're bound to feel overwhelmed and exasperated.

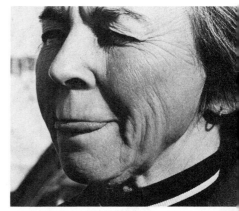

What you do about agitated behavior — whether you meet it in the emergency department, or in some other setting — depends on how dangerous it is. The agitated person who is merely wearing himself out with hand-wringing and pacing may need nothing more than calm reassurance in a quiet environment. However, if he poses a danger to himself or others, he needs restraint. The doctor may order a sedative such as he did with Susan, or some kind of physical restraint.

Whether the patient is mildly or severely agitated, *approach him in a calm, nonthreatening manner*. An agitated patient has a short attention span and will have trouble focusing on anything — so speak to him in short, concise sentences. Such a patient needs to talk about his problem but, since talking about it may make his agitation worse, gear your conversation to his reactions. Allow him some control over the conversation. *Never push him to talk about something if he doesn't want to.* And, when you give information, offer only as much as he can handle.

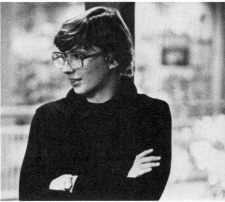

Remember that when an agitated patient becomes assaultive, it may be because he misperceives the situation he's in. Reassure him that no one will hurt him, but that you can't allow him to hurt himself or others. If he continues to act violently, you may need to restrain him physically — and you'll have to make a plan to carry this out. First, determine how many staff members your plan will require and then tell each of them exactly what to do. Approach the patient only after you've organized your plan; never try to restrain him without one.

Working quickly, restrain the patient. As you are doing so, tell him that you've noticed that he's having difficulty controlling himself, and you're concerned that he or others may get hurt. Be sure he understands that the restraint is only temporary. Keep reassuring him and stay with him while he's restrained.

chlorpromazine*	Thorazine Chlorprom◇◇	P.O.: 30-1000 mg daily in divided doses; I.M.-I.V.: 25-50 mg per dose
fluphenazine HCl*	Permitil Modecate◇◇	P.O.: 0.5-20 mg daily in divided doses
fluphenazine* enanthate or decanoate	Prolixin Modecate◇◇	I.M.: 12.5-50 mg per dose
thioridazine*	Mellaril Thioril◇◇	P.O.: 150-800 mg daily in divided doses
trifluoperazine*	Stelazine◇	P.O.: 2-40 mg daily b.i.d.; I.M.: 1-10 mg
haloperidol*	Haldol◇	P.O.: 0.5-5 mg b.i.d. or t.i.d.
thiothixene*	Navane◇	P.O.: 20-60 mg daily in divided doses; I.M.: 8-20 mg daily in divided doses
chlordiazepoxide	Librium◇	P.O.: 5-25 mg t.i.d. or q.i.d.; I.M.-I.V.: 50-100 mg
diazepam	Valium◇	P.O.: 2-10 mg b.i.d. to q.i.d.; I.M.-I.V.: 2-15 mg per dose

*major tranquilizer

Drugs for psychiatric emergencies

The drugs in the table above are commonly used in the E.D. to treat anxiety, agitation, withdrawal from alcohol or drugs, chronic brain disorders, psychosis, neurosis, and psychosomatic conditions. These drugs are classified as major * and minor tranquilizers. Although doctors commonly prescribe major tranquilizers only to treat psychosis, smaller doses of these drugs may be used for conditions normally treated by minor tranquilizers — for example, neurosis, psychosomatic conditions, and mild anxiety and tension.

The symbol ◇ after a trade name indicates that the drug is also available in Canada. The symbol ◇◇ means the drug is available in Canada only. Unmarked trade names are available only in the United States.

Confusion: The case of John Cresswell

You'll probably see confusion more than a few times as you care for patients, because it may result from anything that interferes with normal brain function. Patients like John Cresswell aren't uncommon, particularly in emergency departments.

John Cresswell, a 36-year-old accountant, was brought to our hospital in a state of total confusion. He couldn't walk well or speak, nor did he know where he was or why he was there. Although we weren't able to learn anything about his condition from Mr. Cresswell, his family said that he'd displayed slurred speech during the past 24 hours — also, lethargy, poor concentration and marked disorientation.

When the doctor examined Mr. Cresswell physically, she found no organic cause for his confusion. But when we got a medical history from his family, we learned that Mr. Cresswell had been taking lithium for control of a manic-depressive condition. We suspected lithium toxicity, an increasingly common cause of severe confusion, and ordered a serum lithium level *stat*.

These suspicions were correct. Mr. Cresswell's laboratory

report showed a toxic level of lithium in his blood. He was admitted for lithium detoxification. His only treatment was forced oral fluids to help him excrete the excess lithium. Overnight, Mr. Cresswell's confusion disappeared.

What else can cause confusion? Many things: metabolic and circulatory disturbances, intracranial or systemic infections, cancer, or trauma. Alcoholics and drug abusers may suffer confusion during intoxication or withdrawal. You'll also see it in many elderly patients who are hospitalized, because of their decreased ability to tolerate stress.

Watch for confusion in all patients. It may signal an untreated organic condition that could cause irreversible brain damage. Look for signs of confusion in the way the patient looks, acts and talks:

• Is he unnecessarily disheveled?
• Does he seem dazed, uncertain, or helpless?
• Does he speak haltingly, or in vague terms?
• Is he unable to tell you who he is, where he is, and what's going on?
• Does he nod and say yes to everything you ask?
• Is he unable to follow instructions?
• Does he want to pace or wander about?

A "yes" answer to any of these questions signals confusion for which you must find a cause. Find out from the patient's family what brought on the confusion and when it started. Did some severe psychic stress precede the confusion? Then the confusion probably has an emotional, not organic cause. But if the patient's family report nothing unusually stressful, suspect an organic problem.

Notify the doctor. In such a case, the patient needs a complete physical examination with laboratory studies and a neurological workup.

Here's how to give immediate help to the confused patient. You can group your responsibilities into these four categories: offering reassurance, decreasing sensory stimulation, providing a safe environment, and orienting the patient to reality.

• *Offer reassurance.* Introduce yourself before you speak to the patient. Remember that he'll have a short attention span, so keep your sentences short. Speak softly and calmly; never talk to the patient in a loud or condescending tone.

• *Decrease sensory stimulation.* Take the patient to a room that's quiet and away from activity. Turn on some soothing

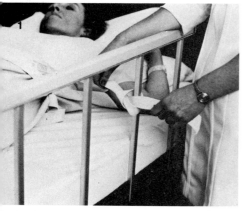
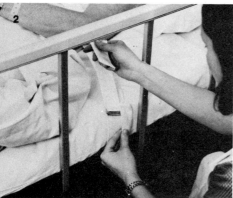

Showing some restraint
If you must restrain your patient, secure the restraints properly so you won't harm him. The restraint in Figure 1 is incorrectly tied to the siderail of the bed. If the siderail were to drop suddenly, the patient's arm could be damaged. In addition, an artful patient could untie the restraint since it would be within his reach. The correct method (Figure 2) attaches the restraint to the bed frame where it cannot harm him or be untied.

music, if possible. Limit the number of people coming in contact with him.

• *Provide a safe environment.* Never leave a confused patient alone; he may wander away and accidentally hurt himself. Many experience illusions; for example, they may see shadows as dangerous animals. Falling out of bed is a hazard; keep the side rails up.

• *Try to orient the patient to reality.* Tell the patient the date and time, and where he is. Explain what you are doing and what to expect.

Never talk about a confused patient's condition in his presence. Remember, he can still hear and understand what you say about him, and deserves your respect. Discourage family members from answering questions you direct at him. His own interpretation of events is more valuable to help you clarify and correct his misperceptions.

Expect to see depression

Some time or another, you'll have to deal with a severely depressed patient — no matter where you practice nursing. You'll recognize him by the sad and downcast way he looks, talks and behaves. Consider depression as a possibility when assessing patients, particularly those who are severely ill. Ask yourself:

• Does the patient complain of tiredness?

• Does he have dark circles under his eyes from lack of sleep or crying?

• Does he sit with his head down and his shoulders slumped?

• Is his facial expression sad? Are his eyes downcast? Does he stare into space? Is he weepy, listless?

• Has he mentioned committing suicide?

• Does he speak in a monotone, in monosyllables, and show no real interest in conversation?

• Does he talk about himself as useless or lonely? Does he depreciate himself?

• Is he passive and unresponsive to his environment?

• Is his sleep or eating pattern disturbed? Has he lost his appetite, or does he eat compulsively?

• Does he seem to have a loss of interest or motivation?

• Does he have difficulty concentrating or completing tasks?

A "yes" answer to any of these questions could indicate clinical depression. *But remember, not every depressed pa-*

tient looks sad and downcast. Some depression hides behind behavior that's agitated and quarrelsome.

What causes depression? We still don't know exactly, but in most patients, the onset of depression follows some catastrophic loss, bereavement, or some threat to self-confidence or self-esteem. The threat may be real or illusory, but could include such things as change in the patient's social, financial, or job status; or a change in his physical condition or capacity to adapt. Traumatic injuries, chronic or disabling disease, surgery or illness — all may represent loss or a threat to some patients. You may also see depression from physiological disturbances, such as acute or chronic brain syndrome, alcohol or drug intoxication, infections, hepatitis or mononucleosis, endocrine disorders (thyroid disease or hypoglycemia), psychosomatic illnesses, anemia, and cancer.

Depression is so common in hospitalized patients that you may have trouble separating the normal mood swings of physical illness from excessive, even self-destructive depression.

Harry Pickering's depression was difficult to spot because he expressed it in behavior that most of us don't associate with the condition. This 72-year-old artist underwent a colostomy for cancer and had to adjust to having a permanent stoma. His adjustment was hampered by a stubborn infection at the stoma site, and soon Mr. Pickering became the most difficult patient on our floor. Fortunately, one of our nurses saw through his unpleasant behavior and got him to talk to her. Soon he began to tell her about his true feelings and fears, especially those related to his surgery and stoma. Mr. Pickering was depressed about his altered body image and feared dying of cancer. His depression had taken the form of hostility — toward us, his family and, of course, himself.

How can you give immediate help to a depressed patient? First, never withdraw from him, no matter how unpleasant he acts. This would only reinforce his feelings of isolation and loneliness. Remember, if you don't give him an opportunity to talk about his feelings, he may find another outlet for them. That outlet could be damaging behavior (as in the case of Mr. Pickering), or excessive complaining.

Establishing a caring relationship is one of the most important things you can do for a depressed patient. In other words, accept him as he is, offer reassurance and hope, and encourage him to express what he feels. Don't become discouraged if this

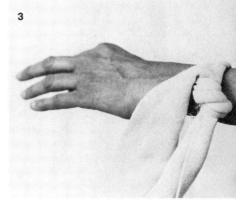

3

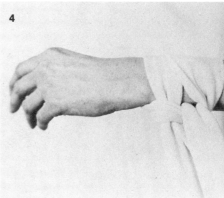

4

Hands down
When securing a patient's hand, do *not* tie a knot in the restraint (Figure 3). If you did, the knot could press into the patient's wrist — impairing his circulation and bruising his wrist as he moved around.

Figure 4 shows the correct method, which allows for movement without constriction or irritation.

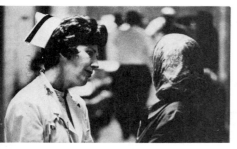

A port in the storm
Working in an E.D. will bring you in contact with emotionally disturbed people who come in off the street. They may be senile and fantasizing; they may be lonely and anxious and make up stories to justify why they are there; or they may merely seek company or a warm place to sit out of the cold. Some you may recognize as repeaters.

Although you know that such cases are not strictly psychiatric emergencies, you must deal with these patients in an appropriate manner. Have a doctor see them or refer them to the hospital's social service department.

isn't easy to do. A patient may reject your attempts—this is his way of expressing his despair. *Caution: Take care while joking with a depressed patient; he may misinterpret your humor and feel ridiculed.* Also, don't be overly friendly; he probably feels he doesn't deserve it.

Watch out for a suicide attempt

Beware of a possible suicide attempt when you're caring for a severely depressed patient, especially if he falls into one of these high-risk categories: he's tried suicide before; he's a psychiatric patient hospitalized for medical treatment; or he became severely depressed in the hospital.

Such a patient may be in imminent danger of suicide if these conditions are present: he talks about suicide; he feels worthless, lonely, or guilt-ridden; he lacks alternatives or support systems; he expresses a need for self-punishment; he's facing a crisis; he's hallucinating; or he's agitated and anxious. Watch for behavioral clues. Has the patient started to "put his affairs in order" or is he giving away prized possessions? Has he told you indirectly what he intends to do through such remarks as "I won't be here much longer." *Caution: Keep in mind that a depressed patient who shows a sudden improvement in appearance and behavior may be in extreme danger.* His improved attitude may only signify internal relief that he's finally made a decision to end his life.

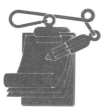

Remember these important points when caring for a patient experiencing a psychiatric emergency:
1. Expect the agitated patient to show physiologic hyperactivity, such as tachycardia, hyperventilation, gastrointestinal distress, and other somatic disorders.
2. Approach an agitated patient in a calm, nonthreatening manner.
3. Never push an agitated person to talk about something he doesn't care to discuss.
4. Beware of a possible suicide attempt when caring for a severely depressed patient.
5. Work to establish a rapport with a depressed patient.

SKILLCHECK

1. Earlier in the day, 35-year-old Benjamin Rhoades was admitted to the hospital with bacterial endocarditis. To combat the infection, the doctor has ordered ampicillin to be given I.M. Before you give Mr. Rhoades his first dose of the drug, you ask if he has any drug allergies. He responds that he is allergic to penicillin. It gives him a rash. What do you do?

2. You are an office nurse in a large suburban clinic. One day, Joseph Wexler, a 62-year-old beekeeper, calls to ask if you can give him the desensitization his allergist has ordered for him. His reason is that he doesn't have the time or the money to keep returning to the allergist for these injections. What do you do?

3. Twenty-seven-year-old Mary McKenna is rushed to the emergency department after splashing laundry bleach in her right eye. She is holding a wet washcloth over her eye and says that she attempted to wipe her eye with the cloth, but received no relief. Mary is very frightened. What can you do to help her?

4. Your city has been hit with the worst snowstorm in its history. You are busy shoveling your car out of a massive snowdrift when you notice your neighbor's car still parked in his driveway. The car is covered with snow, but the motor is running. Working quickly, you clear the snow from the car's windshield and discover your neighbor, a 25-year-old grocery clerk, slumped over the wheel. When you get the door open, you see that his lips and nail beds are cherry red and he has a rapid pulse. What do you do next?

5. Sam Mortenson is a 72-year-old widower who comes to the hospital alone for a suprapubic prostatectomy. He has no preop visitors, because his only living relative — a sister — lives out of state. Immediately postop, Mr. Mortenson is reasonably alert and pleasant to the staff. However, on the third postop day, he becomes confused and agitated. That night, his agitation grows worse and he becomes so disoriented that he forgets where he is. Because Mr. Mortenson repeatedly attempts to get out of his bed despite the side rails and catheter, you use soft restraints to protect him from injury. What else do you do?

6. John Elliot, a 55-year-old corporation president, is admitted to the CCU after suffering an acute myocardial infarction. Unfortunately, Mr. Elliot has been accustomed to having things his own way and finds it extremely difficult to adhere to rules that restrict his activities. He has never before been hospitalized. Not long after Mr. Elliot is moved from the CCU to his own room, he begins conducting business with visitors — as well as over the phone. When restrictions are placed on this type of activity, he becomes argumentative and increasingly upset. Soon, he can't sleep at night. What do you think is wrong?

7. Just two hours after Harry Vanderberg is rushed to the emergency department with a possible myocardial infarction, he develops the signs and symptoms of cardiogenic shock: gallop heart rhythm, narrowing of pulse pressure, a sudden drop in blood pressure, and pulmonary rales. Because you have been monitoring Mr. Vanderberg closely, you notice the change in his condition at once and notify the doctor. When the doctor arrives, he orders dopamine (Intropin) to be given I.V. to increase cardiac output, renal blood flow, glomerular filtration, and urine production. What else should you know about this drug before you give it to Mr. Vanderberg?

8. Mark Conley, a 36-year-old science teacher, is rushed to the E.D. with second-degree burns over 30% of his body area. He suffered the burns in a chemistry lab accident, when the substance he was working with ignited. When you see him, he's alert, his blood pressure is 130/90, and his pulse rate is 96. His respirations are adequate. What do you do next?

(Answers on page 185)

Selected References

American Heart Association. *A Manual for Instructors of Basic Cardiac Life Support.* Dallas: American Heart Assoc., 1982.

American Heart Association. *Heart Facts 1982: A Psychophysiologic Approach.* Dallas: American Heart Assoc., 1982.

American Red Cross. *Cardiopulmonary Resuscitation.* New York: Doubleday & Co., Inc., 1981.

Assessment. Nurse's Reference Library. Springhouse, Pa.: Intermed Communications, Inc., 1982.

Brunner, Lillian S. *Lippincott Manual of Nursing Practice,* 3rd ed. Philadelphia: J.B. Lippincott Co., 1982.

Budassi, Susan A., and Barber, Janet M. *Emergency Nursing Principles and Practice.* St. Louis: C.V. Mosby Co., 1981.

Brunner, Lillian S., and Suddarth, Doris S. *Textbook Of Medical-Surgical Nursing,* 4th ed. Philadelphia: J.B. Lippincott Co., 1980.

Conway, Barbara L. *Carini and Owens' Neurological and Neurosurgical Nursing,* 7th ed. St. Louis: C.V. Mosby Co., 1978.

Cosgritt, James H. *An Atlas of Diagnostic and Therapeutic Procedures for Emergency Personnel.* Philadelphia: J.B. Lippincott Co., 1978.

Dealing with Emergencies. Nursing Photobook Series. Springhouse, Pa.: Intermed Communications, Inc., 1980.

Diagnostics. Nurse's Reference Library. Springhouse, Pa.: Intermed Communications, Inc., 1982.

Diseases. Nurse's Reference Library. Springhouse, Pa.: Intermed Communications, Inc., 1981.

Ensuring Intensive Care. Nursing Photobook Series. Springhouse, Pa.: Intermed Communications, Inc., 1981.

Estes, Nada J., et al. *Nursing Diagnosis of the Alcoholic Person.* St. Louis: C.V. Mosby Co., 1980.

Giving Cardiac Care. Nursing Photobook Series. Springhouse, Pa.: Intermed Communications, Inc. 1981.

Managing I.V. Therapy. Nursing Photobook Series. Springhouse, Pa.: Intermed Communications, Inc., 1980.

Mann, James K., and Oates, Annalee P., eds. *Critical Care Nursing of the Multi-Injured Patient.* American Association of Critical Care Nurses. Philadelphia: W.B. Saunders Co., 1980.

Meltzer, Lawrence E., et al. *Intensive Coronary Care: A Manual for Nurses,* 3rd ed. Bowie, Md.: Charles Press Pubs, 1970.

Moser, K.M. and Spragg, R.G. *Respiratory Emergencies,* 2nd ed. St. Louis: C.V. Mosby Co., 1982.

Moser, K.M., et al. *Flint's Emergency Treatment and Management,* 6th ed. Philadelphia: W.B. Saunders Co., 1981.

Nursing83 Drug Handbook. Springhouse, Pa.: Intermed Communications, Inc., 1983.

Procedures. Nurse's Reference Library. Springhouse, Pa.: Intermed Communications, Inc., 1982.

Providing Respiratory Care. Nursing Photobook Series. Springhouse, Pa.: Intermed Communications, Inc., 1979.

Ramsey, J.M. *Basic Pathophysiology.* Reading, Mass.: Addison-Wesley Pub. Co., 1982.

Sanderson, Richard G., ed. *Cardiac Patient: A Comprehensive Approach.* Philadelphia: W.B. Saunders Co., 1972.

Sokolow, Maurice, and McIlroy, Malcolm B. *Clinical Cardiology,* 2nd ed. Los Altos, Calif.: Lange Medical Publications, 1979.

SKILLCHECK ANSWERS

ANSWERS TO SKILLCHECK 1 (page 25)

Situation 1 — Martin Rogers
Take Mrs. Rogers to a private area and explain why her husband was brought to the hospital. Speak in a calm, low voice and give Mrs. Rogers time to express her feelings. Stay with her for as long as you can and continue to offer her the emotional support she needs. Keep her informed about her husband's condition. Ask if you can phone a relative or friend to come and stay with her during the crisis. Remember, Mrs. Rogers will be understandably distressed about her husband's cardiac arrest. Treat her as you would like to be treated in a similar situation.

Situation 2 — Skip Brennan
Since Skip's friends won't be able to accompany him to the X-ray or treatment rooms, enlist their help in reconstructing the accident. To properly assess the extent of any head or neck injury, you'll need to know exactly how the accident happened, where the patient was injured, and what was done for him immediately afterwards. Once you have this information, you can complete the neurological checklist shown on page 124.

Situation 3 — Mrs. Albert
Obviously, you'll have to postpone treatment for Mrs. Albert's sprained ankle until you can assess the needs of the patients who were injured in the automobile accident. As you do with all patients arriving in the emergency department, check these quickly using the 90-second assessment shown on page 18. When you have completed this and given them any necessary immediate aid, go back to Mrs. Albert and explain what has happened. Inform the other patients who are waiting that there will be a delay.

Situation 4 — Rose Cerutti
Obviously, Ms. Cerutti has reached her emotional limit for coping with stress on this particular day. Chances are, she doesn't really want to quit her job, but just needs some reassurance that her feelings are normal. Be calm and reassuring. Help Ms. Cerutti overcome her distress by showing that you understand her frustration and know how emotionally taxing her job can be. Encourage her to vent her feelings by being a good listener. Tell her how much you appreciate her efforts, and assure her that she is doing a good job.

Situation 5 — Nellie Adams and Valerie Jameson
Take Ms. Adams and Ms. Jameson into a quiet room and tell them what you have observed. Offer them an opportunity to vent their feelings in a nonjudgmental environment. Give each nurse a chance to tell her side of the story. If you are a good listener, you may be able to help them resolve their differences. However, if they can't work together harmoniously after this discussion, you may have to transfer one of them to a different department or put her on a different shift.

Situation 6 — Mary DeVito
As Ms. DeVito's supervisor, you should take her aside and tell her what you have heard. Ask her what duties she expected to perform on her job. Perhaps she has the wrong idea of what her responsibilities would be. On the other hand, Ms. DeVito may just feel insecure about her performance level on the job. If you suspect that this is the case, review her duties with her and assure her that you are pleased with her work. If you are not pleased, tell her how she can improve.

Situation 7 — James Gerhardt
Never expect everyone to respond to stress in exactly the same way. Mr. Gerhardt obviously can't deal with his daughter's tragic death at this moment. He needs more time; his anguish is too great. Be patient, calm, and supportive. Never be judgmental. Watch Mr. Gerhardt's face for clues about what he's really feeling. When he speaks, listen to the sound of his voice; it may reveal more than the words he's saying.

Continue to give Mrs. Gerhardt the emotional support she needs as you work with her husband. Watch Mr. Gerhardt closely. He may require treatment for emotional shock.

ANSWERS TO SKILLCHECK 2 (page 53)

Situation 1 — An elderly woman
The elderly woman may have suffered a cardiac arrest. Working quickly, bend down and shake her shoulders to see if she responds. If she doesn't, quickly roll her over to a supine position and call for help. Look, listen, and feel for signs of breathing as explained in Chapter 3. No evidence of respiration means you must establish an open airway and begin artificial respiration immediately. If the woman does not start to breathe spontaneously after you open her airway, feel for a

carotid pulse. Begin CPR, if needed.

Remember, in case of a witnessed arrest, you can try restoring the victim's heartbeat with a precordial thump. (See Chapter 3 for an explanation of how to administer both the precordial thump and CPR.)

Situation 2 — Virgil Rippy

Just like the elderly woman in Situation 1, Mr. Rippy may have suffered a cardiac arrest. Call him by name and gently shake him by the shoulders to see if he responds. If he doesn't, proceed as you did in Situation 1, with one important exception. Mr. Rippy is a laryngectomee, so you will have to ventilate him using the mouth-to-stoma method. To do this properly, keep the victim's neck level and his head straight. If you hyperextend the neck or twist the head to either side, you could change the shape of the stoma and block the airway. Now seal your mouth around the stoma and blow air in until Mr. Rippy's chest rises. Remove your mouth to allow him to exhale. You don't have to seal off his mouth and nose.

Administer a precordial thump, if needed, and give CPR as explained in Chapter 3.

Situation 3 — Frank Potenick

Do your best to reassure Mr. Potenick — and his wife — during this difficult time. Naturally, you can't be sure his chest pains are caused by a myocardial infarction at first. You'll have to get a complete case history to help the doctor make a diagnosis. Ask Mr. Potenick to describe his chest pains and tell you what he was doing when they started. Follow the other priorities for a possible MI patient, as listed in Chapter 3. 1) Attach Mr. Potenick to a cardiac monitor or EKG machine and obtain a rhythm strip. Then take a 12-lead EKG. 2) Start an I.V. with 5% dextrose in water and, at the same time, draw a blood sample for type, crossmatch, complete blood count (CBC), and electrolytes. Be sure cardiac enzymes are tested; this is especially important when the patient has a possible MI. 3) Keep observing the patient and evaluating his pain as to its character, duration, location, and frequency. Try to assess his anxiety level and administer morphine or meperidine hydrochloride (Demerol) to relieve the pain-ischemia-anxiety cycle, if the doctor orders. 4) Give oxygen by nasal cannula at 6 to 8 liters per minute — or as the doctor orders. Before you do, ask the patient if he has a history of respiratory problems. 5) Get an arterial blood sample drawn to measure the patient's blood gas levels. 6) Continue to give him emotional reassurance and support. Promise that you'll keep his wife informed about his condition. 7) Watch the patient closely and call the doctor immediately if you notice any change in his condition.

Situation 4 — George Baylor

Not necessarily. Sometimes cardiac enzyme levels, when first measured, are normal in a patient with MI. This can happen when he gets to the E.D. quickly; that's one of the reasons you must ask when his chest pain started — it can make a difference. Remember, even though serial enzyme levels can be used to diagnose MI, they're not relied on exclusively. A doctor also depends on EKG findings and information from the patient's case history.

Situation 5 — Jimmy

Ask the guest who is giving CPR to Jimmy to stop momentarily. Reposition Jimmy's airway and resume CPR. If repositioning the airway doesn't correct the distention and Jimmy's not receiving adequate ventilation, relieve the distention by applying gentle pressure over the upper epigastric region. Turn him on his side first, so he doesn't aspirate vomitus. Clear his airway and resume CPR.

Situation 6 — Explosion victims

Using the 90-second assessment as explained in Chapter 1, determine the severity of each patient's hemorrhage by the type, number, and location of the vessels involved. As you know, arterial hemorrhage is always more serious than venous hemorrhage and must be treated first. You can recognize arterial hemorrhage by the way blood spurts out with each pulsation. In either type of hemorrhage, apply direct pressure to stop bleeding and check each patient's vital signs for indication of hypovolemic shock. Estimate the amount of blood lost and record this information on your assessment sheet.

Situation 7 — LeRoy Thompson

Check to see if Mr. Thompson has an open airway and is breathing adequately. If not, open his airway immediately and begin artificial ventilation as described in Chapter 3. Next, remove the towels that are wrapped around Mr. Thompson's arm and try to determine the severity of his injury. Apply direct pressure to stop the bleeding. Now start an I.V. of lactated Ringer's solution and draw a blood sample for a complete blood count (CBC), type and crossmatch, and electrolytes. Use a large-bore catheter so that you can give any needed blood transfusions easily. Check and record his vital signs, palpating both radial pulses. Watch him closely for signs of hypovolemic shock. Examine Mr. Thompson's hand and arm for sensory damage and prepare him for surgery, if needed. Give him emotional support as you assess his injuries and keep his father informed about his condition.

Situation 8 — Jake Justus

Even though his friends' intentions were good, their indiscriminate use of a tourniquet may cost Jake his arm. On the other hand, the tourniquet may have saved his life if they couldn't control Jake's hemorrhage by direct pressure and elevation of his arm. Now that Jake is in the emergency department, evaluate his condition using the 90-second assessment. Start an I.V. of lactated Ringer's solution if he shows signs of hypovolemic shock. Do not loosen the tourniquet; once a tourniquet is applied, only the doctor should remove it. While you're waiting for the doctor to arrive, find out more about the accident from Jake's friends. Ask these questions: When did the accident happen? When did they apply the tourniquet? How long did it take after that for the bleeding to stop? Did they loosen the tourniquet at any time?

If Jake requires a prophylactic injection for tetanus, be sure to first obtain a history of his allergies and reactions to past immunizations.

ANSWERS TO SKILLCHECK 3 (page 79)

Situation 1—Guy Sloane
Mr. Sloane's signs and symptoms suggest pulmonary edema, which may be caused by left ventricular failure. If this is the doctor's diagnosis, he'll probably order the following: oxygen by face mask or IPPB to reverse hypoxia and relieve dyspnea, morphine to decrease ineffective respiratory effort and alleviate anxiety, aminophylline to open alveoli and improve ventilation, digoxin to improve cardiac output, furosemide to promote diuresis, and an EKG to check for recent myocardial damage. If these measures fail, he may also order rotating tourniquets.

Situation 2—Jeffrey Wilson
Check Jeffrey to see if his airway has been obstructed by blood, vomitus, or broken teeth. If it has, remove the obstruction with suctioning equipment or by sweeping your fingers inside his mouth. Do not hyperextend Jeffrey's neck or turn his head to one side, because he may have suffered a cervical fracture. Open his airway with a modified jaw thrust and give artificial respiration, as needed.

Situation 3—Grace Swift
If you give a high percentage (above 40%) oxygen to a patient like Grace, she may stop breathing. A patient with chronic asthma may consistently retain such a high level of carbon dioxide in her blood that the respiratory center in her brain becomes narcotized. Hypoxia, then, becomes her only stimulus for breathing. If you administer a high percentage of oxygen, you can depress that hypoxic drive and cause her to stop breathing altogether.

Situation 4—Christine Shockley
Act fast. Close Ms. Shockley's wound as quickly as possible with a gauze bandage made airtight with a petroleum jelly coating. The best time to apply the bandage is at the end of maximum expiration when

the elevated diaphragm has expelled air and fluid from the pleural space through the wound opening. Hold the dressing snug until the doctor arrives. He'll insert a chest tube to prevent a tension pneumothorax.

Situation 5—Frannie Tighe
Mrs. Tighe's condition has probably progressed to status asthmaticus, and she'll need more aggressive emergency treatment that she's received in the past. Since the usual measures to treat her have failed, the doctor will probably order isoproterenol (Isuprel) administered with an intermittent positive-pressure breathing machine. He may also order a broad-spectrum antibiotic because status asthmaticus may be triggered by severe lung infection. Be prepared to intubate and mechanically ventilate Mrs. Tighe if she goes into respiratory failure.

Situation 6—Joe Delnicki
Don't try to remove the bits of clothing and debris embedded in Mr. Delnicki's chest just yet. Instead, make sure he's breathing adequately and administer artificial respiration, if necessary. Assess the severity of Mr. Delnicki's other injuries and watch him closely for signs of hypovolemic shock.

Situation 7—Neil Erwin
Chances are, Neil has fractured one or more ribs, although you can't be sure until an X-ray is taken. Always suspect fractured ribs in a chest-injured patient when he has pain and swelling in that area, when he tries to relieve the pain by guarding, and when you feel crepitation.

Situation 8—Sarah Espenshade
Always tape chest tube connections firmly to prevent accidental disconnection when the patient is moved. Never clamp a chest tube without the doctor's specific orders, unless the tube gets accidentally disconnected. Make sure the tubing remains patent and does not become kinked or curled. Observe and record the amount and type of drainage from the wound.

Remember, if a major air leak occurs in the tubing while the chest wall is intact—or the tube becomes clogged for more than a few minutes—large amounts of air can accumulate in the chest cavity and cause a tension pneumothorax.

ANSWERS TO SKILLCHECK 4 (page 107)

Situation 1—Gertrude Bingham
Mrs. Bingham's right ureter may have been accidentally incised during surgery. She has some of the signs and symptoms of ureteral injury: pain in the flank and lower quadrant of the affected side, hematuria, and low-grade fever. Notify the doctor at once. Mrs. Bingham will have to return to the O.R. for immediate re-

parative surgery. If urine has already leaked into her peritoneal cavity, Mrs. Bingham could develop peritonitis.

Situation 2 — Margery Vreeland
To help the doctor determine Mrs. Vreeland's condition, as well as the condition of her fetus, take and record her vital signs and listen to the fetal heartbeat. Note the amount of fetal movement, and time contractions carefully. Keep track of the number of pads she saturates and save any expelled clots or tissue for the doctor to inspect. Mrs. Vreeland's bloody show may be due to early labor precipitated by the accident. If labor persists, or becomes more intense, the doctor will probably transfer her to the Ob/Gyn unit. Reassure Mrs. Vreeland and any family members present to relieve their anxiety.

Situation 3 — Thomas Rozecki
Find out all you can about the accident and ask Mr. Rozecki to describe the nature and location of his pain. If his pain increases with movement, is located in his loin or upper abdomen, and sometimes radiates down to his groin or thigh, Mr. Rozecki could have a kidney injury. Since hematuria — frank or microscopic — is also a sign of kidney injury, the doctor will need to catheterize him to complete his diagnosis. Prepare Mr. Rozecki for this procedure and explain why it's necessary. Remind him that catheterization will be less painful if he's relaxed.

Anytime a highly vascular organ like the kidney is damaged, be alert for signs of hypovolemic shock.

Situation 4 — Clare Becker
Mrs. Becker could have an intestinal obstruction, as indicated by her signs and symptoms: increasingly crampy abdominal pain, nausea, vomiting, distended abdomen, high-pitched bowel sounds, and feculent breath. To confirm the diagnosis, the doctor will want you to draw a blood sample to measure hemoglobin, hematocrit, and electrolyte levels. He will also need a urine sample to measure urine specific gravity, and an abdominal X-ray (flat plate). Start an I.V. to keep tissues hydrated and to avoid further acid-base imbalance.

Situation 5 — Sylvia Gibbons
Call the doctor at once. Then take care of the following priorities as quickly as possible: 1) Place Mrs. Gibbons in Trendelenberg position. 2) Start an I.V. with the appropriate solution. 3) At the same time you're starting the I.V., have a blood sample drawn for type, crossmatch, CBC, and electrolyte determination. 4) Take and record vital signs every 5 to 15 minutes. 5) Obtain a complete patient history. 6) Keep track of the number of pads she saturates and save any expelled clots or tissue for the doctor to inspect.

Reassure Mrs. Gibbons and her husband as you work. Remember, they're probably very anxious about her condition, as well as the condition of her fetus.

Situation 6 — Marie Cook
Find out when Ms. Cook had her last menstrual period and ask if she could be pregnant. She has the signs and symptoms of ectopic pregnancy: severe unilateral pain in the lower abdomen, vaginal bleeding, and weakness or dizziness. Notify the doctor, who will want Ms. Cook to come to the hospital as quickly as possible. If Ms. Cook's abnormal pregnancy is not terminated surgically, it could cause a life-threatening rupture with subsequent abdominal infection.

Situation 7 — Bank Guard
The bank guard will probably need immediate surgery to save his life. Call the doctor at once and alert the O.R. Then take care of the following priorities: 1) Cut away the bank guard's clothing, moving him as little as possible to minimize additional bleeding. 2) Start an I.V. of lactated Ringer's solution. Use a large-gauge catheter, so blood transfusions can be given later, if necessary. 3) At the same time you're starting the I.V., draw a blood sample for type, crossmatch, and complete blood count (CBC). 4) Insert a decompression tube to aspirate his stomach contents. 5) Assist the doctor as he inserts a Foley catheter. 6) Reassure the patient as much as possible and explain what he can expect. Ask if he would like to see a priest or hospital chaplain, and call one if he does.

ANSWERS TO SKILLCHECK 5 (page 129)

Situation 1 — Bertha Estus
Tell Mrs. Estus' daughter that she is right; her mother should see a doctor. Her severe unexplained nosebleeds could be caused by a serious underlying disease, such as hypertension or a blood dyscrasia. Or they may be due partly to a drug she is taking, such as an anticoagulant. Get an accurate medical history from Mrs. Estus or her daughter as you attempt to stop Mrs. Estus' nosebleed. To stop the nosebleed, have Mrs. Estus sit down with her head bent slightly forward and show her how to apply direct pressure to her nose with a gauze pad. If this procedure fails, the doctor will probably have to cauterize the bleeding point or apply an anterior-posterior pack.

Situation 2 — Kenneth Markel
Mr. Markel's symptoms suggest that he has a peritonsillar abscess or some other serious throat infection. Naturally, you won't know the diagnosis until the doctor examines him and possibly takes a throat culture, but you do know that some severe throat infections can obstruct a patient's airway. Be ready for this possibility by having a tracheostomy set and suctioning equip-

ment nearby. Watch Mr. Markel carefully for any sign of respiratory distress.

Situation 3 — Anna Malone
Having a buzzing, biting insect in the ear can be extremely traumatic. Assure Mrs. Malone that you can give her instant relief. Then have her sit down and instill a few drops of alcohol in the ear with the Japanese beetle. The alcohol will quickly anesthetize the insect, so you or the doctor can remove it with the appropriate instrument. The doctor may prescribe antibiotic ear drops to prevent a possible infection.

Situation 4 — Donald Hemple
Anytime you assess a head-injured patient you should be prepared in case he has a seizure. If he does, follow these guidelines: Don't panic. Stay with the patient and ask someone to call the doctor for you. Don't waste time searching for a padded tongue depressor for his mouth. Instead, turn the patient on his side, protect him from injury, and maintain a patent airway, if possible. Observe his seizure closely, then record its duration, when it started, which limbs moved, any incontinence, or any unusual posturing. Watch and record the patient's reactions *after* the seizure. The doctor will want a detailed description of all you've observed.

Situation 5 — Buck DeWitt
Make sure Buck has an open airway, and pay close attention to his breathing. If his respirations become rapid and shallow with flaring of the nostrils, suspect trouble. Get help immediately. Buck may require a tracheostomy and possibly a respirator. Since Buck was brought into the E.D. on an immobilization board, let him remain on it while he's getting the needed X-rays. Never try to move a spinal-injured patient unless you know how to do it properly and have enough people to help you.

Situation 6 — Lenny Segal
Obviously, your first priority is to establish an open airway and keep a close watch on the rate and quality of Lenny's respirations. If his breathing changes in any way, notify the doctor immediately. Increasing intracranial pressure from the injury could cause Lenny to develop respiratory distress. If you need to clear his airway, aspirate through his mouth. Nasal aspiration may induce further leakage of spinal fluid, which you have already noted as a complication of Lenny's injury.

How can you be sure the leak is spinal fluid? Test it with Clinistix or use the halo test, as explained in Chapter 12. If you're in doubt, put aside stained linen so the doctor can inspect it.

Since Lenny has a spinal fluid leak, keep his head elevated 30° to put his brain at atmospheric pressure and promote healing. Keep him on absolute bedrest in the correct position. Instruct him not to blow or pick at

his nose, and cover his ear with a gauze pad, so it can drain naturally.

Situation 7 — Leslie Davenport
Most likely, Leslie has a fractured larynx. She has all the signs and symptoms of this injury: severe face and neck pain, difficulty swallowing, loss of normal voice, swelling, and crepitation. To give her the proper emergency care while you're waiting for the doctor to come, follow these guidelines: 1) Prepare for possible airway obstruction. Have a trach set and suctioning equipment nearby. 2) Check vital signs frequently and watch Leslie for signs of respiratory distress. 3) Never leave her alone.

ANSWERS TO SKILLCHECK 6 (page 179)

Situation 1 — Benjamin Rhoades
Don't give Mr. Rhoades the injection of ampicillin, because it is a penicillin derivative. If you did give him the drug, he could have a serious allergic reaction — for example, anaphylactic shock. Instead, find out more about the reaction Mr. Rhoades had to penicillin. What kind of rash was it? How long ago did it happen? When you have recorded this information on his chart, ask about any other allergies that Mr. Rhoades may have and make sure the doctor is notified.

Situation 2 — Joseph Wexler
Ask the doctor if you can give Mr. Wexler his desensitization injections. If he says "yes," tell Mr. Wexler that you will need a letter from his allergist ordering the serum and outlining the treatment plan. Inform the patient that he must bring the serum in a properly labeled bottle with complete information about the amount and frequency of dosage.

Before you give Mr. Wexler any injections, make sure you have oxygen and emergency drugs (epinephrine and antihistamines) ready in case he goes into anaphylactic shock. Never permit the patient to leave the office until you have observed him for at least 20 minutes after each injection.

Situation 3 — Mary McKenna
Hold Ms. McKenna's right eyelid open and thoroughly irrigate her eye with water, using an I.V. tube. Have her lie on her right side when you do this, so you don't wash the chemical into the other eye. Call an ophthalmologist immediately so he can evaluate any damage that may have been done to Ms. McKenna's eye.

Situation 4 — The neighbor
Pull your neighbor out of his car into the fresh air. Most likely, he's been overcome by carbon monoxide when the snow clogged the car's exhaust pipe. Establish an open airway and begin artificial respiration immediately. If you see a passerby, tell him to call an

ambulance and inform the dispatcher that the victim will need oxygen. If no one is nearby, wait till your neighbor is breathing adequately and make the call yourself. Cover him with a coat or blanket to keep him warm.

Situation 5 — Sam Mortenson
Before you fasten the restraint, make sure that Mr. Mortenson's bladder is not distended and that his catheter is patent and draining adequately. Check him closely for early signs of septicemia or any other condition that may be responsible for his distress. If you can't find any physical cause for Mr. Mortenson's confused and agitated behavior, call his sister and ask her to give you a more complete patient history. He may have had episodes like this before.

Situation 6 — John Elliot
Mr. Elliot may be using a denial mechanism to cope with his illness. This is a very common response in patients who have suffered an MI. Chances are, Mr. Elliot has great difficulty adjusting to his sick role. He's accustomed to being in control of his life and now others seem to be controlling him. Talk to Mr. Elliot about this, if you can, and try to get him to express his feelings. Involve him in making more decisions about his care. For example, help him find a way to structure his day so he can meet some of his needs within prescribed limitations.

Situation 7 — Harry Vanderberg
If dopamine (Intropin) infiltrates surrounding tissue, it can cause sloughing and necrosis near the injection site. To prevent this, start the I.V. in a large vein — preferably one in the antecubital fossa — not a vein in the hand, wrist, or ankle. If drug infiltration occurs, stop the infusion immediately and call the doctor.

Depending on his response to dopamine, Mr. Vanderberg may need his dosage adjusted. If his blood pressure elevates excessively, his dosage may have to be reduced or discontinued. Watch for wide swings in blood pressure and check for fluid overload. Stop the drug immediately if he develops headache, chest pain, premature ventricular contractions.

Situation 8 — Mark Conley
Make sure Mr. Conley has an open airway and provide humidified oxygen at a measured volume. With a large-bore catheter, start an I.V. to give lactated Ringer's solution and serum albumin. See that a Foley catheter is inserted to monitor Mr. Conley's urine output. Get an arterial blood sample to measure blood-gas levels, take vital signs, and give further burn care as explained in Chapter 14.

Index